All the Difference

All the Difference

a memoir

Patricia Horvath

Etruscan Press

Etruscan Press
Wilkes University
84 West South Street
Wilkes-Barre, PA 18766
(570) 408-4546

W
WILKES UNIVERSITY
www.etruscanpress.org

Published 2017 by Etruscan Press
Printed in the United States of America
Cover artwork by Jeffrey LeBlanc
Cover design by L. Elizabeth Powers
Interior design and typesetting by Susan Leonard
The text of this book is set in Warnock.

First Edition

16 17 18 19 20 5 4 3 2 1

Library of Congress Cataloging-in-Publication Data

Names: Horvath, Patricia, author.
Title: All the difference / Patricia Horvath.
Description: First edition. | Wilkes-Barre, PA : Etruscan Press, [2017]
Identifiers: LCCN 2016054248 | ISBN 9780990322191 (paperback)
Subjects: LCSH: Horvath, Patricia--Health. | Osteoporosis--Patients--United States--Biography. | Osteoporosis--Popular works. | Self-care, Health--Popular works. | BISAC: BODY, MIND & SPIRIT / Healing / General. | SELF-HELP / Personal Growth / Success.
Classification: LCC RC931.O73 H68 2017 | DDC 616.7/160092 [B] --dc23
LC record available at https://lccn.loc.gov/2016054248

To protect the privacy of actual people, some of the names in this book have been changed.

Please turn to the back of this book for a list of the sustaining funders of Etruscan Press.

This book is printed on recycled, acid-free paper.

To my mother, who was there.

She is still asking herself where this body ought to be, where exactly to put it so that it will cease to be a burden to her.

—Marguerite Duras,
The Ravishing of Lol Stein

Acknowledgments

Excerpts from this work first appeared in *Cream City Review* and *2 Bridges Review.*

I wish to thank the New York Foundation for the Arts, the Barbara Deming Memorial Fund, Hedgebrook, Millay Colony for the Arts, and Blue Mountain Center for their support. Thank you, as well, to Framingham State University.

For their encouragement and sage critique I thank Robert Dow, Marita Golden, Michelle Hoover, Jane Rosenberg LaForge, Jeffrey LeBlanc, Jay Neugeboren, Kate Southwood, Elizabeth Fairfield Stokes, and Michelle Valois. Thank you to my mother, Maureen Cotter, and to my brother, Howard Horvath, Jr., for putting up with my questions. Thank you to Chris Bullard for his sharp editorial eye. Finally, thank you to the good people at Etruscan Press, most especially Bill Schneider and Pamela Turchin, for their belief in this book and their hard work in helping it come to fruition.

All the Difference

Patricia Horvath

Prologue

I may as well admit it, I'm poorly put together. My body leans sharply to the left. I'm brittle-boned, stoop-shouldered, with an "S" shaped spine. I cannot touch my toes, ice skate, or ride a bike. My right shoulder blade and hipbone stick out too far, and my right leg is a half-inch shorter than my left. When I walk, my right foot swings wildly to the side. On its own trajectory, my foot will skim the sidewalk's detritus: potato chip bags, stones, bottle caps. My ex-boyfriend called it my "trick foot." We'd pass, say, a dented car or battered-looking hydrant. Look what the trick foot did! he'd exclaim and I'd laugh, wanting to be a good sport. It's important to be seen as a good sport when one is, in fact, completely unathletic.

Dry Bones

The doctor was "astounded."

Patient suffers from marked osteoporosis, the report read. *Fracture risk is high. Treatment, if not already being done, should be started.*

He told me the results did not make sense. "You have the bones of a seventy-year-old. Are you sure you don't smoke?" "Never." "And . . . you're definitely still menstruating?" "As we speak," I replied. What I wanted to say was "See? You should have believed me!" because for nearly two years I'd been insisting to skeptical doctors that I was shrinking.

Two years earlier I'd been living in Massachusetts, finishing up my MFA degree while teaching sections of freshman composition at two different schools. On a typical day I got up around seven, made a pot of coffee, and drank it over the course of several hours while I wrote, then headed to my grad courses in the late afternoon. Tuesdays and Thursdays I taught morning classes at a state college and afternoon classes at my university. Either way, sometime around noon I'd rush through a meal of yogurt and fruit. Dinner was just as perfunctory—defrosted soup, maybe a sandwich. Weekends I wrote and graded and looked for jobs. Some nights I met up with other grad students at readings or bars where we drank beer and listened to music and talked about life after graduate school, which in my case would entail a move to Harlem and an adjunct teaching job. The job would eventually grow into a full-time position, but I could not know that then. Meanwhile,

I drank too much coffee, ate too little, exercised infrequently, and all the time I was slowly shrinking. I could not know that either.

Because I was graduating, and losing my health insurance, I decided it would be a good idea to get a check up. Aside from intermittent bouts of insomnia, which I'd had since adolescence, I felt fine. Nevertheless, one morning in late May I took off my shoes and stood on the doctor's scale. I've always derived a certain goofy pleasure from these check-in rituals. The nurse straining on tiptoe to record my height. Or nestling the larger of the scale's two weights into the one hundred pound slot then sliding the smaller weight too far to the right and having to guide it back—slowly, slowly—well to the left of where she'd started. The inane, jocular comments: My you're a tall drink of water! And: I bet you can eat whatever you want.

This time, though, the nurse barely had to stretch. She rested the level against my head and wrote down a number—sixty-seven inches. But sixty-seven inches was wrong.

I'm five-eight, I said, startled. The scale's not right.

It's a scale.

She picked up the blood pressure cuff, waiting for me to roll back my sleeve. Other people were waiting too—a room full of patients she had to weigh and measure. This nurse was a busy woman who did not have time to indulge her patients' whims. Still, she relented. I stood up as straight as I could. I pulled back my shoulders and lifted my chin. The vertebrae in my spine cracked as I tried, uselessly, to will them to straighten. I stretched and stretched to my full height . . . five foot seven.

But last time—I began.

You can discuss it with the doctor. Now let's look at that blood pressure.

In the doctor's office I changed into a crinkly paper gown. The day was unseasonably cool; I could feel goose bumps rising on my arms. I wanted my coat. I wanted to go home, get my coat, start the day over. Come to think of it, if I'd really shrunk an inch, why did my coat still fit? And my other clothes, few of them new. Shouldn't my pants be dragging the ground, my sleeves dangling?

I thought of my father's mother, hunchbacked and tiny by the end of her life. Didn't I take after her—birdlike in a family of big-boned people? She'd been diagnosed with osteoporosis, the "widow's stoop," as it had then been called. I knew the risk factors, knew they were against me: a small-boned Caucasian woman, dwelling in a northern climate and living the sedentary life of a graduate English student who'd just spent the past year teaching seven courses at two different schools while working on a book. A woman who, as a child, had loathed milk and spent her summers reading indoors. Someone whose biggest treat had been a trip to the library—not the children's library, but the adult one where the floor was made of glass bricks lit from below and the book titles were not, I understood, to be taken literally but instead held mysterious, hidden meanings. My grandmother and I spent hours in the stacks. She craned to reach the higher shelves. We were alike in more ways than one. Still, she was my *grand*mother, old before I was born. Women my age weren't supposed to shrink.

The doctor came bustling in—smiling, pleasant, visibly harried. She apologized for keeping me waiting, and she began to ask about my general health.

I'm shrinking, I interrupted. I think I have osteoporosis.

She looked at me, clearly puzzled. I'd been seeing this doctor for years. She was thorough, calm, a good listener. We'd commiserated about issues of women's health: the needless difficulty, say, in attaining the "Plan B" morning-after birth-control pill or the nearly instant FDA approval for Viagra while RU-486, the French "abortion pill," had been banned by the FDA for over a decade. So I was genuinely taken aback when my doctor told me no, this could not be, I was far too young to have osteoporosis. A baseline bone density exam would be conducted at the onset of menopause, perhaps another ten years. How short, I wondered, would I be by then?

I could feel a small rip opening at the back of my gown as I shifted in my seat. My thighs stuck to the hard plastic of the chair seat. I wanted to get on with the exam, but I knew I was not leaving until she took me seriously.

I've shrunk an inch, I said.

The doctor looked through my file. She had no record of my height. My last measurement must have been with my previous doctor, at least three years earlier. Perhaps, she suggested, that scale had been inaccurate? Perhaps I was mistaken?

I'm a shy person, soft-spoken. I dislike confrontation. On the subway, if someone vacates a seat, I'll look around to see if anyone else needs it before sitting down. If a student comes to me upset about a grade, I'll listen to her arguments. Sometimes I even change the grade. But this was different. This woman, my doctor, was standing between me and my health. Because the insurance industry or medical profession or whoever it was who makes these decisions had determined that women my age could not have osteoporosis, women my age were not tested for the disease. How then could I support my claim?

I told the doctor that I needed her to authorize a bone density exam. She refused, saying that premenopausal women are not at risk for osteoporosis. But my mistrust of my body—too profound for her words to sway—convinced me I was right.

Look, she said, it's highly unlikely you have osteoporosis.

Highly unlikely or impossible?

The doctor opened her desk drawer, took out her prescription pad. Patients were backed up, waiting to see her; not yet noon, it would only get worse. We hadn't begun my exam. She wrote something down and, unsmiling, handed me what I needed.

When the results came back, she called. The doctor said she was sorry for having doubted me, it was good I'd been so insistent. Still, I had to understand how unusual this was. I felt vindicated, but also angry. Not only at the doctor, but at myself. Why hadn't I noticed that in three years no one had recorded my height? Wasn't I the one ultimately responsible for my health? If I'd paid closer attention . . . then I stopped. How else could I have known? I had to shrink to realize that I was shrinking. I hung up the phone and began to cry. You're my doctor, I wanted to shout. What if I had listened to you?

Femur, tibia, fibula—I pictured the long bones in my body crumbling to powder. The doctor had mentioned Fosomax. I'd seen the commercials: silver-haired women rode horses and did leg lifts at the ballet bar while an announcer intoned *See how beautiful sixty can be.* As far as my doctor knew, no studies had been conducted about the long-term effects of Fosamax on forty-year-old women. She'd called an endocrinologist at Massachusetts General Hospital who'd told her that Fosamax can remain in the bloodstream for up to seven years. Supposing I became pregnant?

The doctor recommended exercise, calcium, Vitamin D, a follow-up visit in a year. It was nearly two years, however, before I had health insurance again. This time I knew exactly what to do. I made certain I was measured. I'd shrunk another quarter inch. When my new doctor balked (Osteoporosis? Are you sure?) I had proof. Now, with a fresh batch of results showing further bone loss, he was "astounded."

He said it was essential I start taking Fosomax. He also set up an appointment with an endocrinologist at St. Luke's Roosevelt Hospital near Columbia University. Late winter, early spring I walked from my apartment in Central Harlem past the decaying buildings along Frederick Douglass Boulevard, through Morningside Park, up the hill to Amsterdam Avenue, where the neighborhood abruptly turned cleaner, shuttered buildings giving way to bookstores and cafés, welcoming beneath bright awnings. Snow melted to mud, crocuses poked through the earth, then daffodils, tulips, until the park was a riot of new growth.

The endocrinologist—British, exceedingly polite—ordered tests. Lots of tests. I had blood drawn twice, another bone density scan. For twenty-four hours I peed into a jug that I lugged back to the lab in a plastic Fairway bag. The next day I got a call—they'd neglected to give me a vial of preservatives to mix into the jug; I'd have to redo the test. Up and down the hill again with my jug of urine. When the tests finally came back, they revealed nothing—except that I had osteoporosis. The endocrinologist confessed to being "perplexed." But I was not. My bones have always been treacherous, and once again they had betrayed me.

Testifying

I moved to New York during the first year of the new century, a boom time, though my neighborhood, Central Harlem, was not yet booming.

The sales office for my building was a double wide trailer parked on West 116th Street. The marketing director, a formidable woman with a crown of coiled braids, referred to me as her "queen." As in: "And how is my queen today?" Like the other women in the office she was overtly religious, and on the day I signed the purchase and sale agreement for my unit, a Sunday, she celebrated by inviting me into the office staff's prayer circle. I stood between her and the accountant in a group of a dozen or so praying, swaying women, all of us holding hands. Some of the women "testified"—about struggles overcome, family members who needed help, a son in prison, a daughter with an addiction, a diploma recently achieved, people who needed prayers of supplication or thanks. I didn't know the words to the prayers and I had no inclination to testify, but I felt moved to be included in this circle, to have crossed some invisible barrier from client to communicant. When it was my turn to give thanks, I said simply, I'm so happy to be here.

Across the street from my new building were two vacant lots heaped with demolished car parts that glittered in the sun. The lone neighborhood supermarket had brown lettuce, sawdust-strewn floors, gangsta rap. There were abandoned buildings on both sides of every block. Crack vials crunched underfoot; I had to pay attention whenever I wore sandals. But my apartment was large and sunny, and every day, weather permitting, I went for a walk in Central Park.

I had only to read the paper to be reminded, starkly, of how my neighborhood differed from New York below 110th Street. There, people ate gold-flecked desserts in celebrity restaurants. Hermès kept a waiting list for five-figure Birkin bags. A famous woman with a famous father backed her Mercedes SUV into a crowd of people milling about a Hamptons nightclub while screaming "Fuck you, white trash!"

I'd known about the excess before moving, of course. Still, the contrast between where and how I lived and the antics taking place to the south was jarring. One day, I no longer recall where, I read an article about a couple who had plastic surgery and liked the results so much that they decided to have their children undergo the process, too, "So we'll look more like a family."

I'd been diagnosed with osteoporosis only a few months earlier, and it occurred to me that this was a serviceable metaphor for the creative person in the consumerist vortex that was twenty-first century Manhattan. So I wrote a story in which a woman, a poet, is shrinking so rapidly that she has to carry a milk crate to stand on. When she disappears entirely, no one notices.

The story, being somewhat heavy-handed, didn't really work. It was funny, but tainted by bitterness. I knew that. Still, I showed it to some colleagues in my writing group, who asked me about the piece's genesis.

So I told them. About my osteoporosis and then, haltingly, about its precursor, scoliosis, the years I'd worn back braces and body casts, my spinal fusion at age fifteen, the difficulty I'd had re-learning how to walk, the even greater difficulty of learning to see myself as "able-bodied."

I'd known these women for years. We'd gone to grad school together, had met every Thursday night for dinner and workshops, and had stayed in touch when school ended.

They were astonished. We had no idea, they said. Why didn't you ever tell us?

It doesn't seem important anymore. Even as I said this, I knew it was a lie, a way of distancing myself from the house of cards I still felt my body to be.

That's the story you need to write. They were adamant and unanimous.

I didn't want to listen. These women, my confidantes, were urging me to open a door I'd nailed shut. No, I thought, I'll never write that; it's nothing I want to revisit.

But I knew they were right. Without vexation, another word for conflict, there's no story. I'd held back for so long, erased so many years. Difficult as it might prove, maybe writing would be a way to reclaim them. The next day I began.

Tests

I'm straddling my red Schwinn bike, from which the training wheels have been removed. My mother holds onto the fender, steadying me. For nearly an hour I've been trying unsuccessfully to balance. I am eight years old, past when the training wheels should have come off. Younger kids, my six-year-old brother among them, are already whizzing around our cul-de-sac. Chipper keeps circling by on his orange two-wheeler with the banana seat. He's gone from taunting me to shouting encouragement, realizing, I suppose, that something just isn't right. Ready? my mother says, Keep peddling! She lets go. For two, three seconds I manage to stay aloft, then the bike wobbles and I skid on the asphalt, skinning my hands and knees. I struggle to my feet, and this time I do not pick up my bike. Let it stay there, let it rust. I go inside, find a book. I will try again, try all summer, before giving up entirely.

In elementary school I quickly learned that what matters occurs *outside* the classroom. On blacktops and playing fields, alliances formed. The race really went to the swift—and social prominence too. But I got tangled in jump ropes, couldn't hit a ball, ran races too slowly (my right foot heading in a different direction altogether from the rest of my body). Sports were an impossibility; I didn't even like to watch. Unless the game was basketball, where my height was an asset, I resigned myself to being last picked—the scrub choice. I was shy, uncoordinated, a socially awkward girl voted "Most Likely to Succeed" by sixth grade classmates who, like me, had little notion of adult success. I told myself being last didn't matter. Eventually we'd return to the classroom where the team captain could barely stutter his way through a paragraph and the blacktop queen would flub the spelling bee. After school, though, no one rushed outside to play Spelling Bee.

The difference between my own shortcomings and those of my classmates seemed to me largely a matter of exposure. If someone flunked a test, that was between her and the teacher. No one posted the scores. But my lack of coordination was on display every single day. I felt this distinction keenly, never more so than during the annual Presidential Fitness Test.

This was actually a series of tests—chin-ups, push-ups, high jumps, sprints—most of which I failed. Each year I knew I was going to fail; my classmates knew it too. What I resented was the prominence accorded the tests—the theatrics of them, the applause for high scorers, the exhortations of our gym teacher with her stopwatch and bully's whistle, her back slaps and admonishments. *Don't be a baby! Toughen up!* Her formula was simple: tough kids aced the test; babies flunked.

I panted through races where I came in last. I clung to the chin-up bar, trembling, unable to hoist myself level. I toppled sideways trying to do cartwheels and forward rolls. And for what? At the time Lyndon Johnson was President, then Richard Nixon. I couldn't picture either of them—the jowly cowboy, the shifty-eyed man with the raised shoulders—mastering even a single cartwheel, let alone the entire test. Yet each had become the most powerful man on earth. How much did fitness really matter?

The kids who could chin themselves repeatedly, hit homers, and run fast—where were they running to? Every night on CBS Walter Cronkite intoned the number of dead. Those who could not touch their toes or who were smart enough (and fortunate enough) to get into college were spared. The "tough kids," blacktop bullies, had no use for books. They excelled at all things physical, and this was their time. But who, I wondered, would applaud these high scorers once they'd grown up?

Books

They did not fail me. They opened new worlds and kept the existing one at bay. Books were my fortress; I could hole up inside of them. Better than that, they were portable. I brought books everywhere: summer camp, Sunday drives, errands with my mother, even the bathroom.

I read the usual suspects: Hans Christian Andersen, the Brothers Grimm, *Black Beauty*, Louisa May Alcott (whose *Little Women* made me cry, but whose *Little Men* I finished only from a sense of duty). I read indiscriminately. Dickens of course and Aesop and the *My Book House* series from my mother's childhood with their elongated yellow and black illustrations of fairies and elves. But also Archie comic books, Bazooka Joe bubble gum wrappers, my grandparents' *Reader's Digest*, ("I Am Joe's Kidney," "Grizzly Bear Attack: Drama in Real Life") and an entire gothic series about a family named Falcon that lived under a curse borne down generations by its female members, who were moody, beautiful, and extravagantly wicked. Weekends, summers, school vacations, I stayed in my room reading. If I were being punished, my mother would send me to Chipper's room, where the only things to read were a children's encyclopedia set, some *Mad* magazines, and a book about football. I read those, too.

My favorite book was *D'Aulaires' Book of Greek Myths*. Every week during fourth grade I checked it out of the school library except for one brief period when the librarian made me stop, insisting that I needed to give the other kids a chance to read it. For weeks the book stayed on the shelf, out of bounds, until, sick of my pestering, the librarian relented.

I loved the Greek gods. Their violence and glamour and pure weirdness topped anything in the Bible or on TV. They rode dolphins, wore winged sandals, turned themselves into animals. I lived in a world of banal heroes: flying, punching comic book figures with their masks and capes—Batman, Superman, Spiderman—boy heroes like Underdog with his simpering girlfriend, Sweet Polly Purebred; sports heroes who made my father jump up screaming from the couch during weekend games. On sitcoms there were heroines: genies and witches who yearned to be housewives. So what if Jeannie and Samantha had magic powers when all they wanted—all women were *supposed* to want—was to wash dishes and make beds?

The Greek goddesses, though, had no desire to stay on Mount Olympus baking pies. My favorite was Athena. Goddess of wisdom and the arts, she'd sprung fully formed from Zeus's head. No one told her what to do and no one dared mock her. Just look at what she'd done to poor Arachne, shrunken to a spider for disparaging the gods. Yet Athena was not casually cruel like Artemis, nor jealous like Hera, and she certainly didn't lose her head over men the way Aphrodite did. Not only that, she carried an owl on her shoulder and wore a breastplate made from Medusa's severed head. I wanted to be just like her. *D'Aulaires' Book of Greek Myths* said she had gray eyes; mine were blue-gray, close enough. I pretended our cat was an owl and tried to balance her on my shoulder, which didn't really work. I wore belts with giant buckles, imagining they were the Medusa head. One cross word, one dirty look, and I would turn my tormentor into stone.

Reading whetted my appetite. The more I read, the hungrier for words I became. In books, too, I found an inherent sense of justice, the triumph of the downcast. Andersen's duckling may have been ugly, Oliver Twist abandoned, Jo March eccentric and poor, yet somehow they prevailed. The scorned, the deformed, the misunderstood, I rooted for them all. And, inevitably, I began to wonder about their creators. Someone had crafted each book I read, crafting in the process a writer's life. Eventually it occurred to me that this making of books was a serious thing, a way of reshaping the world.

I began to write as randomly as I read: journals, lyrics, odes to nature, fairy tales, stories about girls overcoming all types of adversity. Aside from school assignments, I kept my writing to myself, suspecting, perhaps rightly, the perplexity it would cause my family. No one I knew wrote; why on earth would they? The adults I saw did serious, practical work. The women taught school or worked in beauty salons or as secretaries. The men had more exciting options. My father, who worked as a private detective, kept a gun in a shoebox on his bedroom closet shelf. I'd discovered it while rummaging through my mother's dresses and wigs. I imagined car chases, shoot outs with bad guys, all kinds of glamorous things to write about. The gun scared me, and I never told anyone I'd found it. But when I asked my mother in a roundabout way what, exactly, my father did for a living, I was disappointed to learn it had nothing to do with chasing bad guys and instead involved something called "insurance fraud" and (I later learned) the occasional wandering spouse. It was impossible to imagine the adults I knew hiding in some attic like Jo March or Hans Christian Andersen, chomping on apples and thinking about things. Besides, there were hardly any books in our home. True, my grandmother made weekly trips to the library, mostly for mysteries, and, true again, my mother's parents had a huge stack of *Reader's Digest* magazines. But the biggest collections of books in our extended family belonged to me.

My mother, while proud of my grades, worried about my increasing isolation. She urged me to go outside and make friends the way my brother did. Athletic and affable, Chipper collected friends like I collected, well, books. Nearly every week he'd come home from school with some new classmate. They'd ride bikes, make cardboard forts, shoot marbles, flip baseball cards—none of which interested me. Once in a while, though, because they were younger, I could cajole them into playing some game of my own invention. We'd play Circe and I'd turn them into swine. Or Dream

Game, in which I'd have everyone pretend to sleep while I acted out my dreams of the previous night. These games never lasted long. My brother and his friends got tired of being transformed into livestock or having to snore on command. Your sister's games, they complained, are really stupid.

One afternoon, fed up with the way I "moped around the house," my mother made me call up a girl who lived two streets away. Squat and loud, a nose picker who never read anything at all, the girl repulsed me. Do it! my mother said, holding out the receiver. Do it or you can spend the entire week in your brother's room. I'd already read everything in there including the baseball cards. So I caved. The neighborhood girl and I spent a desultory hour or two playing Barbies until I managed to fob her off on Chipper, who was always happy to have another kid around. Then I snuck off to my room to read.

Silence

All the students in Mrs. Satler's classroom, even the tough kids, knew to keep out of her way.

On my first day in this new school I was assigned the last seat in a row of alphabetized fifth-graders, one of several exactly spaced rows, so different from the "open" classroom I'd attended the previous year. There we'd been encouraged to ask questions and "work at your own pace." Fridays had been "casual" days; girls could wear pants. Nothing doing in Mrs. Satler's classroom: *Girls, you will be young ladies.*

Earlier that year my father had moved out, the private eye shacking up with his secretary, and we'd gone to live in my grandparents' house in a new school district. Mrs. Satler emphasized discipline, obedience, conformity. That first day, she read the roster in a voice that belonged to a bird of prey. She called each student by his or her full name—*Patricia Lynn Horvath. We do not use nicknames here!* On the coldest mornings she kept us outside. We stood shivering in our separate lines, boys and girls, stomping our feet, our faces hidden behind scarves and hoods, our eyes and noses streaming. To the right and left other students greeted their teachers and were let into their warm classrooms. We waited. Eventually Mrs. Satler would come to the door.

Good morning class, she'd recite flatly.

We looked at her. What kind of day would it be?

Good morning, Mrs. Satler, we'd reply loudly, in unison, cold air in our throats.

What? I can't hear you!

GOOD MORNING, MRS. SATLER!

Is that the best you can do? In that case, you can all stay out there and freeze! And she would slam the door.

One day she grabbed a boy by the hair and, laughing maniacally, pushed his head into his locker. Another morning she whipped off her wig and waved it at us. April Fools, she screeched. I'm bald! Even the boys quieted, and a girl burst into tears. I knew that at night Mrs. Satler's human shape fell away and she assumed her true form—the Medusa.

Mrs. Satler ignored her No Nicknames rule whenever it suited her, which was most days. I was "Sieve Head," an honorific awarded me the day I forgot some homework assignment. Some kids, mostly boys, she hit with rulers. One or two girls she made pets of, praising their work, letting them erase the board. She was especially partial toward a Scandinavian looking girl named Nelsa who was embarrassed by this and used to tell the other kids, during recess, It's not my fault, I hate her too. Because she was pretty, and uncomfortable with her status, no one held it against her.

I pleaded with my mother to let me stay home. I told her about the wig, the locker, the name-calling. She complained to the principal, but so did the other parents, all of them demanding that their child be transferred to the other fifth grade class. Mrs. Satler had us write letters. The theme: Why You Hate Me. We could, she said, remain anonymous. Still, we lied. She read the letters aloud. *You're a nice teacher. We don't hate you. Sometimes you're a little mean*—here she lowered her glasses—*but mostly you are nice.* My mother later told me Mrs. Satler submitted these letters to the principal. Whether the ruse worked or whether it was something else, she remained in her job until she elected to retire.

Sixth grade was no better. Every morning Miss Swenson read to us from *Pilgrim's Progress.* The pilgrim wandered a bleak landscape, beset by sin, while we fidgeted, itchy in wool sweaters, the gray sky hard against the window, the language of the story impenetrable. We memorized poems that were never discussed. One by one we stood to recite "O Captain! My Captain!" Walt Whitman,

I decided, was a sailor, a famous captain's son. His father had collapsed on deck (heart attack?) and now he was sad.

For hours we practiced penmanship, Miss Swenson's leathery bicep jiggling as she drew cursive letters on the board. She had us copy long passages from our science text: *That'll teach you to be sloppy. I hope you all get writers' cramp!* One of her favorite pedagogical strategies was to pit students against each other. She'd select a piece of work she considered exemplary: a drawing, a story or poem. *Look at that shading! Listen, how imaginative! Why can't the rest of you do that?*

The drawings often belonged to a girl named Joyce, and the writing was usually mine. We'd lower our heads, knowing what was next:

Now look at this. Someone's NOT EVEN TRYING!

Miss Swenson tore drawings in two. Read stories aloud, mistakes and all. Looking back, I believe one of her favorite targets had dyslexia. She'd read his work ("dog" for "God," "angle" for "angel") while he sat at his desk, turning red.

Recess was payback. The kids who were mocked in the classroom vented their frustrations the minute they were let outdoors, insulting those who could not race, jump, or kick, shunning the awkward and slow. Unable to compete, I stayed apart, watching, wishing the teachers would let me read. I did not want to be Miss Swenson's star pupil, Mrs. Satler's joke. Hiding in corners, keeping my mouth shut, seemed the safest way of avoiding these twin dragons. If no one noticed me, no one could single me out.

I'd always been shy in school, but in this new environment I kept a monk's silence, only speaking—whispering, practically—when spoken to. Sometimes not even then. I waited for the day to wind itself down so I could go home, where I felt safe enough to have a voice. I was hoping teachers and students alike would give up, leave me alone. It almost worked.

Each week the guidance counselor, a matronly woman, pigeon-breasted in frilly polyester blouses, pulled three girls from our sixth grade class. One of the girls had been kept back at least once and was already growing breasts. Another sat vacantly, twirling her long blonde hair and giggling. Both these girls were frequent victims of Miss Swenson's ridicule. The third girl was the one who had cried the year before when Mrs. Satler tore off her wig. All three were in the slow reading group. Mid-year the guidance counselor came into our room, the same as always, and went up to Miss Swenson's desk. She whispered something; Miss Swenson pointed. I slouched in my seat. The guidance counselor beckoned. I pretended not to see. She walked over to my desk and told me to come with her. From that day on, I was part of her special group of girls.

At first I thought it was a mistake. These were the slow girls, the ones in remedial reading and math. I was quiet, not stupid. Couldn't they tell the difference? Furious, I refused to participate. I sat in the circle, but would not open my mouth. I vowed to work harder, get straight A's, show everyone that I did not belong.

Earthbound

Sometime during the spring of sixth grade, the gym teacher sent me home with a note. She'd noticed how off-center I appeared when trying to touch my toes. Perhaps, she wrote, our pediatrician should take a look. A week or two later I stood in the doctor's office in my underpants, bending over, raising my arms, shifting left and right, while he measured arms and legs, shoulders and hips. I leaned forward, arms dangling, knees straight. Touch your toes, he said. I couldn't, the only kid in my class unable to do so, but so what? It wasn't like I couldn't read. Why, all of a sudden, should this require a doctor's visit? I was bad at sports, that was all. Soon I'd put on my clothes, take a lollipop from the fishbowl on the receptionist's desk, and go home. But the doctor asked me to sit down. He told my mother and me that I had scoliosis—a double, S-shaped curvature of the spine—and referred us to an orthopedic clinic at Bridgeport Hospital.

On our first visit to the clinic I sat in the waiting room, a long corridor with welded-together chairs that faced each other from opposite walls. Many of the patients were young girls like me. Some wore elaborate-looking back braces that made them sit up rigidly, their necks restrained behind stainless steel bars, their chins thrust forward onto plastic podiums. Several wore leg braces; one girl had a prosthetic leg that ended in a clunky brown shoe, like something an old man might wear. A few people seemed normal enough, though God only knew what they (or I) might look like coming out of the doctor's office. For once not even a book could distract me.

I was not entirely certain what had landed me in this place. My spine was curved, that much I knew, my right side shorter, thwarted, out of all alignment. The word *scoliosis* meant little to me. I'd flunked a lot of fitness tests. I had a funny walk. Could they put you in the hospital for a funny walk?

There were many patients, one doctor; the wait, I discovered, could take all afternoon. When the nurse finally called my name, I trailed her and my mother into the examination room. My mother helped me tie the blue cotton gown in back. She looked me in the eye when the doctor would not and politely rephrased his third-person questions ("How does she sit?" "Honey, how do you sit?") until he took the hint and asked me directly.

I lay on the examining table and the doctor measured my legs. I bent over while he took a protractor to my spine. I stood on one foot then the other. It was a game of Simon Says. The doctor muttered as he wrote things down. I was the body in the room, there yet invisible.

That day I was x-rayed for the first time and saw what a misshapen thing my spine was. It started out straight enough but about a third of the way down, my spine began a dramatic curve to the left, making an "S" shape as my lower vertebrae snaked back in the other direction before managing, somehow, to merge into my tilted pelvis. It was a wonder, I thought, that I could stand at all.

Dr. Mangieri explained that I had idiopathic scoliosis. I hated that word, *idiopathic*, the way it sounded like *idiot*, suggesting some causal link, some malfunction not only of body but of brain. Was this why I'd been lumped in with the slow girls in guidance? What did brains have to do anyway with a crooked spine? Later my mother explained to me that idiopathic meant the cause of my curvature was unknown. For scoliosis, this was common. Left untreated, the doctor continued, my condition could lead to progressive deformity, chronic pain, possible damage to pulmonary and cardiac function. My translation went something like: This is serious, pay attention, do what he says. And what he said was to exercise. Because I was still growing, he felt that a physical therapy regimen would strengthen my back muscles, helping them prod my spine in the right direction. If that didn't work, I would have to wear a brace. And if that didn't work . . . But on that first visit I don't think he brought up surgery. What I remember is that the threat of the brace turned me into a physical therapy zealot, willing my muscles to straighten my recalcitrant spine. I would not become like those girls in the waiting room, a spectacle encased in plastic and steel.

To correct the half-inch imbalance in my leg length, I would have to wear a shoe with a built-in lift. The lift was expensive and the shoe had to be sturdy. In the dawning era of platform heels, I started junior high with two pair of orthopedic shoes—sensible brown oxfords and saddle shoes. They were heavy things, nothing like Hermes's winged sandals. They made me feel earthbound, and I loathed them.

Good Girls

Twice a week I went to physical therapy. Because my mother worked, she arranged for her mother to pick me up from school and drive me to the rehab center.

My grandmother built her week around these excursions. A few years earlier she'd left her beauty parlor job and had begun a quick slide into a whiskey-fueled retirement. When my parents divorced she let us have the house and moved to a one-bedroom apartment, which she and my grandfather uneasily shared. She slept until mid-afternoon, gulped down handfuls of brightly colored pills with an orange juice chaser, then fixed herself the first in a long string of Manhattans. Most days she didn't bother to get dressed. Sometimes though, when we stopped by for a visit, she'd be wearing the longline bra girdle-garter belt ensemble that meant she was going out. This she kept partly concealed beneath an open robe, a modest touch. The garment, with its hooks and straps and elastics, fascinated me. My grandmother wore it whenever she had errands, most often a trip to the pharmacy for cigarettes. Was this, I wondered, what old women had to do to leave the house? My mother wore normal underwear—bra, panties, an occasional slip. My father's mother, who wore stockings and white cotton gloves even in summer, wouldn't dream of showing her underwear. Did she, too, wear one of these things? Would I have to?

My grandmother sat on the couch, feet up, tissues, cigarettes, and drink in reach. She smoked Newports by the case, two packs a day, coughing her way through conversations, railing against the doctor who'd told her to quit, triumphant when he dropped dead of a heart attack. *Doctors—what do they know?* And she'd gesture toward my grandfather, silent and unmoving in his La-Z-Boy. Had doctors been able to cure his Parkinson's disease? She'd fix herself another drink.

Squat and pugnacious, my grandmother cherished a fight. She needed an antagonist, someone around whom she could build a dramatic narrative. Her sons-in-law—the deadbeat, the bully. The neighbors with their yapping dog. The paperboy who always came late. And the Tomlinson Junior High School crossing guard who had the nerve to expect her to park in the visitors' lot when her granddaughter had a medical condition and needed to get to therapy and how the hell difficult was *that* to understand?

From high up on the school steps I'd see her, vivid in a paisley dress, her gold Camaro first in a line of idling buses. *Bet the other kids think your grandmother's pretty cool, huh, driving a Camaro. Bet they wish they could come too.*

The longer I waited on the steps, the greater the commotion. My grandmother always parked up front, ahead of the buses, which, she pointed out, had plenty of room to maneuver around her. This was true. But she was up against a Rules Are Rules crossing guard who, like her, was convinced of the moral rightness of his stance.

The crossing guard wrote a citation. My grandmother tore it up. Buses honked. My classmates watched. I was certain that my great love Señor Raul, the handsome young Spanish teacher with the red Corvette and the 007 license plates, was watching, too. Señor Raul who—from what misguided impulse I cannot say— slipped me love notes in the halls: *Patricia, mi amor, mi corazon.* No, I wanted to holler, this woman with the lacquered hair and gold car, the one waving her arms and shouting, no she did not belong to me. But she did and, chastened, I scurried over to the car, sinking low in the passenger seat.

It's okay, I'd say. You can park around back. I'll find you.

And get caught in that traffic? We have to get you to therapy. You have a medical condition—I told him so! Trying to make me go around back. We pay taxes! Who the hell does he think he is?

On and on it went. I put a textbook up close to my face until we were out of school range.

In rehab the other patients soaked in whirlpools or practiced using walkers. They bragged about grandchildren and complained to their therapists about their aches and pains. My therapist was a brisk woman with a German accent and a husband who'd run into trouble with the local Board of Education for barring girls from his high school shop class after the law changed to let them in. The therapist claimed these girls were troublemakers who did not know their place. I, on the other hand, was a good girl, meaning I did not care about shop. By confiding in me, the therapist implied that she and I were conspirators, united in our disapproval of these willful, boyish girls. Never did it occur to her that I might recoil from the idea of being limited and defined by one's body. Years later, when her husband was at last fired for discrimination, I was glad.

The therapist and I worked on "balance and resistance." I walked a wooden beam, inches from the floor. I lay on my stomach, trying to keep my arm raised while the therapist pushed against it. Gut girl! she'd cry, encouraging me. But I did not want to be a good girl. I did not want to take shop, I did not want to lie on my stomach behind some therapist's partition of curtains, I did not want to wear orthopedic shoes. I wanted to be David Bowie, whom I'd recently discovered on FM radio, or Twiggy, whose glammed-out face appeared on the cover of Bowie's album *Pin Ups.* I wanted a different body, no body, an elongated body like the one I had, all jutting bones, elbows, clavicle, only different. A body that would land me on the cover of an album rather than a therapist's table.

The therapist gave me exercises to do. Every night, for twice as long as she specified, I practiced with the headphones on, listening to Mick, to Bowie. Or I practiced to Cher's variety show—another one-name wraith with attitude. As I did my arm lifts and push-ups, I imagined myself onstage, a back-up dancer shimmying in glitter.

I am a tightrope walker, see me so lithe. Arms outstretched, school-books piled by the high curb in front of the Mobil Station. Toe, heel, toe, heel . . . steady. It's not easy to be agile in these shoes; three times this week I've crashed to my death. Chin up, don't look down, ignore the spectators—my fans—pumping gas, wiping windshields, digging for change in their pockets. My foot slips, misses the curb, and I tilt dangerously, flailing my arms. Close! But this time I make it, all the way to the end, hopping down with a twirl of my invisible parasol. The gas station attendant applauds, embarrassing me, but I am pleased, too. See what I have done!

Once a week our seventh-grade class met with the guidance counselor, who showed us movies about drugs. Drugs would make us hear voices, kill ourselves. Look at Diane Linkletter, daughter of the TV show host. She'd taken some LSD then jumped out a window. We saw a filmed reenactment of this and another educational movie in which a young man takes an assortment of mismatched pills and winds up in a hospital. His voice, in halting monotone, told of his experience: *It was three weeks before I could remember my name.*

These movies were overwrought, hard to take seriously, but the etiquette films were worse. One, about how to date, starred a very young Dick York, the first Darren from *Bewitched.* With his bug eyes and wide white part, that nasal voice, we recognized him right away, the boys in class chanting "Durwood." Here he played a teenager who trolls around his father's garage fixing antique radios. Concerned, his father tells him to swap his suit jacket for an argyle sweater, "act natural," and start meeting girls. Another film, on the do's and don'ts of dating, depicted the travails of a young man named "Woody." Woody makes a mess of things, mashing his poor date at her doorstep as she cries "No, please!" This, we were informed in voice-over, was *Wrong! Let's try again.* This time Woody mumbles "Well, so long," abandoning his befuddled date at the door. Finally, Woody gets it right. He tells his date he had a great time, promises to call her next week, says good night—without the two of them touching.

It was ridiculous. A kid named Woody. The guy from *Bewitched*. We'd seen Dick York turned into a monkey, a werewolf, seen his ears grow to the size of feet. What was our guidance counselor thinking? In retrospect, though, the movies had a message, one that we couldn't help but absorb: boys act, girls wait to be acted upon.

I began eighth grade the tallest girl—nearly the tallest student—in my class. A couple of important things had happened over the summer. First of all my mother had remarried. Her new husband was a short-tempered short man, a Nixon Republican, fervent drinker, and junior partner in his brother's law practice. He could tolerate Chipper, but as for the bookish, sullen adolescent who'd suddenly taken up residence in his home, he made it quite clear that he'd just as soon I find somewhere else to live. Except when absolutely necessary, Tom and I did not speak to each other for the twelve years he and my mother were together.

Another big change had occurred that summer: my growth spurt. I'd gained nearly two inches since seventh grade, much of it over the summer. As I grew, my spine became more twisted. I could feel the curve, the wayward vertebrae just beneath my skin. My hipbone stuck out so much that when I wore low cut jeans, I looked all out of proportion. My right sleeve hung lower than my left; I was always pushing it back. And in school, my right shoulder blade knocked against my chair, bone chafing metal. No matter how I shifted in my seat, I could not get comfortable.

I was still going to physical therapy, but I was slipping by degrees. Every three months I returned to the orthopedic clinic. The routine was always the same. Wait in the corridor outside the examination room. Change into the thin blue gown, then wait in a cubicle to be x-rayed. The x-ray room buzzed with machinery like a low, persistent headache. I would lie on the table and hold my breath as the machine passed over me. Right side, left side, hips hard against the table. Then the table would be tilted upright and I'd do another set, standing.

The doctor began to scowl almost as soon as he switched on the light table. He drew white lines on the films, measured angles of curves, compared current and previous x-rays, and the comparison was never good. For over a year I had been exercising daily and going to therapy twice a week, but by the time I entered eighth grade, it was clear that this was not enough. My spine now looked to be on a collision course with my left hipbone. The doctor explained that I would need to wear something called a Milwaukee brace, a chin-to-hip plastic and metal apparatus like the ones I had seen girls wearing in the clinic waiting room. The brace, he said, would prevent my scoliosis from getting any worse, but would not reduce the severity of the double curve. I would live in this carapace for twenty-three hours a day, seven days a week, until I stopped growing, which he estimated would be in three years. The doctor explained all of this in his customary technical language. Beyond the raw details (brace, twenty-three hours a day, three years) I don't think I took much in. Questions? he asked, but I had none. His sentence was final; it brooked no appeal. He switched off the light table, and my illuminated spine disappeared.

Caged

We drove to a place near the overhead tracks for Amtrak and Conrail. If you were to take the train through Bridgeport now, thirty years later, it would look much the same: piles of tires, car parts in abandoned lots, scabby triple-deckers—an abandoned, broken place.

My mother parked the car, locked it, and led the way to a storefront with prosthetic limbs in the window. There were walkers, bedpans, corsets, canes, all dusty. I did not want to go in. I may have said no, may have said let's turn around, I may (more likely) have acquiesced. The brace—like the exercises, the orthopedic shoes, like fitness tests, mandatory friendships, and my mother's remarriage—were all things to be endured.

We were greeted by a large, stubble-faced man who was smoking a cigar. He was the maker of these corsets and limbs, a man who would spread his tobacco-stained fingers on my torso, breathe his sour breath into my face. Dwarves came into the shop, cripples, amputees. He put his hands on them, too, gave them new limbs.

The man told me his name, Buxbaum, said he was going to put me in traction to make a plaster mold of my torso. My mind flashed to a black and white commercial from my childhood. Seat belts! an elegant woman complained. They're so inconvenient, and besides, they wrinkle my dress. Ominous drum roll, quick cut to an accident victim (the same woman!) in a head-to-toe cast, her limbs suspended by pulleys from the poles of her hospital bed. Traction.

I must have blanched. In any case, the brace maker tried to reassure me, saying it wasn't so bad. By now I knew enough to know that "not so bad" meant at least somewhat bad and probably worse than that. We went into a back room that was like an auto mechanic's garage, only with braces and limbs instead of cars. Scattered about were all sorts of tools: saws, chisels, wire clippers, things I did not recognize. The room was drafty and cold. I undressed behind a flimsy wooden partition with a metal stool for my clothes, keeping on my underpants and socks. The floor was dirty. The brace maker wrapped my torso in gauze then strapped my head into a sling. He hoisted me up with a pulley until I was hanging by my chin, my toes barely touching the grimy floor. My hands gripped two monkey-bar-like handles for support, but my weight was all in my chin.

Buxbaum whistled as he stirred a large plastic bucket of plaster. His breath was rancid and there were moth holes in his cardigan. Each layer of plaster had to dry before the next one could be applied. With each new layer, the corset heated up and pressed harder against me, making it difficult to breathe. I hung by my chin, trembling. My jaw ached. I tried shifting the weight from my chin to my hands, but I was strapped in too tight. I couldn't speak, so I moaned. How much time passed I could not say. When Buxbaum finally freed me, cutting the corset loose with a giant set of shears, I just about collapsed. My jaw was so stiff I could not move it. Bits of plaster clung to my skin. I got dressed, feeling soiled.

In school I didn't tell anyone I would soon be wearing a brace. Being solitary, I didn't have confidantes, and I doubt, in any event, that I possessed the ready language for such a conversation. I didn't want anyone feeling sorry for me or teasing me or making a fuss. I was glad to be excused from gym; other than that, I suppose I was hoping to go unnoticed.

I spent the days before my brace was ready in a kind of countdown state. Three more nights of sleeping "normally," I'd tell myself. Two more days before everyone knows. One more day of freedom, one more day to be just another girl.

The hard plastic corset buckled in back with a thick leather strap. Attached to this new torso were metal suspenders. I stepped into the brace, put my arms through the suspenders, and grabbed the dresser for support. My mother tugged and tugged. The strap was heavy; it had no give. This was her first attempt at shackling me, and she was having trouble. The corset bumped against my hips. I sucked in my stomach. My mother pulled harder on the strap. I was a debutante being corseted for the antebellum ball. She gave one final emphatic tug and the brace shifted into place on my hips. I could feel the strap buckling, a screw being tightened at the back of my head. I looked at my reflection, looked away. This was me now—these metal bars, these bolts and screws. I pulled up my jeans, but they wouldn't fit over my hips. My shirt was too tight to button.

The brace's weight was incredible, a second body to lug. I was tall and slim, but caged I was a heavy, clunky thing. The corset made me stick out in back. I needed pants large enough to fit over my plastic torso, shirts that could accommodate my metal shoulder blades. But my limbs had not grown longer. My new, double-digit sized clothes were too long in the leg and arm. My mother spent evenings hemming, but do hemmed jeans ever look right?

Shirts were especially difficult. The brace had numerous gadgets and straps. One white strap cut across my abdomen, another attached to the bars just above my clavicle and would peek out from low-necked shirts. Even in summer I wore turtlenecks and scarves. The material had to be thick or it would shred against the brace. Eventually my shirts sported balding patches at the right shoulder blade; these would give way to tiny holes. I loved glitter, gauze, Indian prints. I wore flannel, smocks, cotton pullovers. I rolled the sleeves back so they would stay. My earrings clicked against the brace's metal neck ring, so I gave those up too, trading them in for gold "starter" posts.

Sleeping was the most difficult thing of all. The neck ring and molded plastic rest at the back of my head prevented me from lowering myself directly onto my pillow; instead I made a mound of pillows, high and soft enough to sink into. If I rolled over during the night, the weight of my brace often woke me. I slept intermittently, beginning a lifelong struggle with insomnia. I turned on the bedside lamp and read deep into the night. Blue crescents formed beneath my eyes. I became sluggish—what did it matter, I could barely move. A soap-bar shaped piece of plastic pressed continually into the small of my back. Since I couldn't bend, I needed to sit in straight-backed chairs. I could not look down, nor see in any direction except straight ahead unless I turned my entire body. The metal desk-chairs at school provided little support—an oval back rest maybe eight inches high, an armrest for right-handed students only. To read or write I needed to lean far forward in my chair. My right shoulder blade chafed against its suspender, becoming red and sore. The corset left welts on my hips. Like a car, I would periodically check into Buxbaum's garage for "adjustments" but I never felt adjusted, not for a single day.

The idea of a brace "fitting" is in a sense anomalous, as the purpose of a brace is to mold the body to its own contours. My right hip protruded too far, my chin not far enough. Alternately I would thrust my chin forward onto the chin rest or tuck it against my neck to avoid the offending piece of plastic altogether. Doing so, I pictured myself a turtle, retreating into its monstrous shell. But I also felt safer, less exposed. Because I was constantly on display. Children pointed. Old women, my grandmother's friends, clucked sympathetic sounds. Strangers felt free to question me: *What's that thing for? How long do you have to wear it? Do you sleep in it?*

At meals I could not bend to my plate, but had to raise my utensils level to my mouth. I made messes. My mother's husband complained. Eating became unpleasant; besides, the corset sat heavily on my stomach. I ate small portions, skipped breakfast and lunch. Were it possible, I suppose I would have shrunk myself small enough to disappear entirely, slithering like Houdini from my shackles.

But in another sense, I was already invisible. For what people saw was the brace, not the object locked up inside. There are metaphors for this. Rapunzel, Sleeping Beauty—the princess imprisoned in the fortress. Snatched from the world by some calamity, she whiles away her youth, unperceived and unperceiving.

I thought about this and rejected the metaphor. I did not see myself a damsel in distress. But the male gaze—is there any force more potent to the adolescent girl? The messages we received through television, advertisements, fairy tales, movies, music— especially music—encouraged us to define ourselves in its beam. Mick sang "Under my thumb," Robert Plant sang "Shake for me, girl," Steven Tyler sang "Beg for my big ten inch." The boys in school were gawky and gross. They punched each other and belched; they made rude noises. Still, we were told, they and their older brothers mattered. A girl unremarked on by boys suffered more than a lack of stature. In a sense she ceased to exist.

Though I was cloistered, I was not the damsel in distress, the sweet, coveted thing. For one thing, I was too angry—full of silent "fuck yous" from morning till night. And then, well, there was the physical fact of me. Sleeping Beauty did not have a crooked spine. Rapunzel did not wear a brace. Either one could likely have elicited an appreciative belch from a fourteen-year-old boy. I was, however, locked away like them, subject to some awful power beyond my comprehension. Extending the metaphor, did that make my mother the witch? I suppose I must have thought so. After all, it was she who locked me in at night after my shower, that one-hour slice of freedom I enjoyed. She whose job it was to keep me caged:

No, you may not go to the beach, take it off for So-and-so's party, yes, I know it's difficult to sleep, but.

How she must have hated that role. Trapped between the warring needs of her husband and daughter, stubborn creatures both, unwilling to bend, she now had the added burden of enforcing my confinement. I wheedled and begged: *One half hour more, let me sleep without it, just tonight, look at this rash, my skin can't breathe, c'mon!* I raged: *Why do I have to wear this stupid thing, so what if my spine's a little crooked, who cares?* I was sullen, resentful; I was thirteen and did not know how to make things easy even in easier times.

Recently, in a manila envelope stuffed with old family photographs, I came across a yellowed sheet of paper, typed on both sides and folded into quarters. I thought it must be some ancient draft of a story I'd abandoned and, curious, I began to read:

I feel the urge to write about the fears, anger, comic moments, and joy we experienced and hope this story may strike some familiar chords or help those about to face a similar situation.

An intelligent girl, shy in school, demanding at home, Pat at thirteen had too many adjustments to make at once. Adjusting to my remarriage, adjusting to junior high school, and adjusting to wearing a metal brace from hip to neck. Just when boys and awareness of her body loomed large on her horizon, POW, the doctor stuck her in a shiny metal contraption. The worst affliction that can occur to an adolescent: to be made to appear "different." It didn't help that I made allowances too often for these problems.

This was the opening to an English paper my mother had written some thirty years earlier for a university night course.

My mother hates to write. She'll barely email. On the rare occasions she has to compose something more complicated than a thank you note, (the last occasion being a letter to the editor of her local paper) she'll call me to ask if I'll look over her notes, fix things up, make them sound "elegant." Invariably she'll hand me something that sounds like her own voice: thoughtful, articulate, immediate. The kind of voice many writers—myself included—struggle to attain. You're a natural, I tell her but No, she says, it's just too plain.

Knowing this, I can sense how difficult this paper must have been for her to write. Words are crossed out, typed over. Shorthand symbols and abbreviations are penciled in the margins. The page resembles a neater version of my own heavily edited drafts. Toward the end, the draft devolves into a series of fragmentary notes: *Mention friends. J.* Given the topic, my mother's attempts to frame her thoughts on paper would have been particularly fraught.

As I read, I felt increasingly uncomfortable, as though I were invading my mother's privacy. And it was unnerving to see myself presented so bluntly in someone else's narrative. (Of course I plead guilty to mining the lives of family and friends; as a writer that's my "job.") Yet this is my mother's story, too. I found the writing compelling for the insight it shed onto her perspective. What were these "joys" she mentions? I survived to write this piece, using past tense verbs. (*We lived through it*, she writes, *that is enough.*) By including me in the plural pronoun, she implicates me in her point of view. But the joy I recall occurred much later, when I was once again able to feel the sun on my body, sleep through the night, sit without pain. It was the joy of release. What, I wondered, were the "allowances" for my "problems" that my mother felt she made? How did she see this time? How did she manage?

I filed the paper in a folder with my medical records and the notes I'd begun to accumulate about causes and effects of scoliosis. Among other things, I'd discovered a link between spinal curvature and bone disease.

Bones, of course, are strengthened by exercise, calcium, Vitamin D. Once braced, I was excused from gym. I became lax about physical therapy. The whole point, as I saw it, was to prevent me from being braced, so why bother? I ate little, stayed indoors. The brace's metal parts heated quickly in the sun. I sat out summers in my air-conditioned bedroom. I read and studied more than ever, made the Dean's List, getting A's even in subjects I did not like. If I could not be a body, I would be a brain, nothing less, nothing more.

I'd begun my research in a state of uncertainty. I knew by my doctor's initial reluctance to authorize a bone density test that I was "different," that I fit into some minute category that encompassed my brittle bones, my crooked spine, my wayward walk; that these impairments heightened my natural tendency toward introspection and solitude, a rejection of things physical which, in some circular fashion, had put me at risk for bone loss. I was angry at my bones. Why *not* lose them; they'd given me so much trouble? Why not become a brain in a jar or, better yet, a sprite—Ariel, Tinkerbell, Quisp the Cartoon Martian, androgyne, nearly bodiless, completely free? I had so many questions—about the nature of disability, about the body/mind dichotomy, about how disability shapes identity and what happens to that identity when physical difference disappears. Writing let me grapple for answers. I wanted to understand why I broke down crying when my doctor told me I had bone disease. Her diagnosis had made me feel vulnerable and afraid. Why was this so threatening? How had my experiences with scoliosis shaped my reaction—shaped, in a larger sense, the person I had become? These were the things I wanted to discover.

I decided to mention the English paper to my mother and tell her what I was working on. This, I knew, would not be entirely easy. I'd made a decision to dwell on a difficult period of my life, difficult not just for me, and now I wanted to drag my mother back there, to glean whatever insights she might have, use her memory to prompt my own. It was, I realized, a selfish decision and yet it felt essential.

Allowances

My mother has no memory of the English paper. When I show it to her she peers at the yellowed sheet, turning it over, running her finger along the heavily penciled notes. Then she refolds it, returning the past to me.

What does this mean? I ask. You made 'allowances.' What 'allowances?'

Oh, honey, she says. That was so long ago. You had a lot of . . . issues. A fresh mouth. Stubborn. People—Tom, my mother—said I spoiled you, let you have your own way too much. They didn't try to understand. You were so unhappy—who wouldn't be?

As much as possible, I avoided my mother's new husband. His dislike made me nervous. When he entered a room, I would leave. When his car pulled into the driveway, I would go upstairs. Sometimes, though, I wouldn't hear the car. I'd be in the den, deep in stereo fog, listening to Led Zeppelin or the Stones. Eyes shut, headphones clamped tight, I'd startle as the dial spun to the EZ Listening station. Without a word, Tom would yank the headphones from the jack and walk away.

At night I could hear them. *She's thirteen. You're the adult. She's in a brace, can't you just?* And Tom's words—*attitude, straighten up, spoiled.* From an economic perspective, I suppose that was true, I suppose I was spoiled. Because my mother had married an attorney, the son of a judge, we were no longer struggling, no longer a household headed by a single woman with a high school education. To help me sleep in the brace, my mother had bought me an air-conditioner. Later I would have my own phone, appointments with orthopedic surgeons at elite hospitals, private duty nurses, new clothes to fit my changing shape as I went in and out of braces and casts. It was my mother who paid for these things, but she was able to do so only because someone else now paid the mortgage and covered our household bills. As an adolescent, I never really stopped to consider this, never thought about how much worse things could have been without Tom's income to soften my physical discomfort. Overnight we'd gone from scarcity to plenty. I took our new status and the things it bought for granted. What was money for if not to live well?

My mother bought me a stereo, one with bubble speakers, albeit no headphone jack. Music was one of the few things that took me out of myself, and she let me play it louder, I suspect, than if I hadn't been braced. Her new husband believed in rules, deference, bedtimes. I'd never had a bedtime. So long as I remained on the Honor Roll, my mother didn't care when I went to bed. "Sack Time, USA!" Tom would proclaim night after night. I'd glance at Chipper contemptuously as he scurried into his pajamas. He wanted to be liked. I wanted to watch *Don Kirshner's Rock Concert*—downstairs, on the color TV. I stayed where I was. Tom spoke white noise, words I did not heed. My mother, I knew, would back me up.

For Christ's sake. Let me raise my own kids!

They fought about family. About politics, money. Unlike Tom, my mother had grown up poor. Her mother had left school at fifteen, going to work in a dime store after her father was fatally scalded by a laundry room boiler. During the Depression, she picked cherries on a Michigan farm. My mother's father joined the Navy right after high school. It was the GI Bill that vaulted him and his young family into the lower reaches of the middle class. Early in my grandfather's life his parents divorced and he spent his childhood moving from rooming house to rooming house. He'd come home from school to find the boxes packed, his mother one step ahead of the landlord. My grandfather's job was to carry the family's lamp.

My mother, too, spent much of her childhood moving: Milwaukee, San Francisco, San Jose, Brooklyn, Long Island, Bridgeport, wherever her father was stationed. After the war, they moved from Brooklyn to a prefab housing development on Long Island. Little shitboxes, my grandmother called these houses. She hated Long Island—the soggy potato fields that were slowly being drained and parceled into suburban lots, the look-alike homes, the lack of transportation, the long walk into "town," which was little more than a general store and a post office. To make things worse, her husband was soon reassigned to the naval base in Boston, increasing her sense of isolation.

This was when her drinking began in earnest. My grandparents separated, sending their two daughters into foster care with families that ranged from indifferent to hostile. My mother and aunt lived out of suitcases in strangers' spare bedrooms. When, after nearly three years, their parents reconciled and my grandfather was reassigned to Panama, the entire family went with him. By now my mother was entering high school, a bright, vivacious girl who loved parties and clothes. She had two skirts and three blouses—all sewn by her mother.

It was in Panama that the first tremors of my grandfather's Parkinson's disease began. A taciturn man, he confided to my mother that he was afraid—something was happening that he did not understand and could not control. He put in for a transfer and was reassigned to a desk job in Bridgeport. It wasn't long before he was unable to work, taking early retirement and disability pay.

Meanwhile my grandmother swung into action. Her youngest child, born after the reconciliation, was starting school, her oldest graduating, no reason to stay home. She got her GED and began studying for her beautician's license—manicures, pedicures, leg waxing—practicing at night on my mother. They were a family of five in a two-bedroom house. My mother shared a room with her sister. Their brother slept in the upstairs hallway and the girls had to walk through his "room" to reach their own. (Years later my brother would sleep in this same hallway, outside my bedroom, my mother's old room.) There was one bathroom.

At night, home from her job cashiering at the A&P, my mother would help make dinner. Each night the same. Her brother, hungry, wanting to know when he can eat, who will go over his homework. Her mother with her feet in a bucket of Epsom salts. Tired from standing all day, she's downing a Manhattan. The table needs setting. Her sister—where is her sister? Has she borrowed a scarf again, a favorite sweater that she will return soiled? Perhaps my mother has a date, is in a hurry. She hadn't asked to be the oldest, to have to do these things. Her father's speech has become slurred, difficult to decipher. His shuffling gait. It will not get better.

The chance of my mother going to college was zero. College was where you went to get the skills you needed to support a family—something women did not do, despite the fact that my grandmother, and later my mother, wound up doing precisely this. My mother was smart. She liked school. But school was ending. She took a job as secretary to a salesman in a firm that manufactured machinery to seal tin cans. That salesman, Geza Horvath, had a son. My mother met him at a Christmas party and within six months they were engaged. She was eighteen, he twenty-three.

Eventually she would wind up back there, the home she left for one of her own. She would take another secretarial job. Support from my father would be promised—later mandated—but it never quite managed to arrive. Doctors' bills went unpaid, rent was late, groceries were a juggling act of sales and coupons and supermarket fliers. Somehow I knew this, information being one of the dubious advantages that accrue to the inconspicuous child. But there were also clues. It might have been the homemade clothes, or the way certain words—"restaurant," say, or "vacation"—took on a reverential tone. The way we were told *No, I'm sorry, you can't see your father until . . .* Or, *You're not sick enough to stay home, do you think I can miss another day?*

Once in a while she talked about moving. Only where would we go? I could almost feel her thinking . . . *What next?*

Money was a problem and then abruptly, with my mother's remarriage, it was not. No, that's not quite right. Money was a problem, but in a different way. Only one person in our new makeshift family of four had money. Three did not. And that one never let the other three forget.

My mother's new husband, youngest child of a judge, had one job his entire life: junior partner in his brother's law firm. The open door, the Vacancy sign, the smile obsequious and eager, these were familiar to him. During his childhood his parents had a maid, took cruises, ate in French restaurants where the maitre d' knew their names, sat them at the best tables. He'd attended prep school, a Jesuit seminary for boys. Sometime during the fall of his senior year the guidance counselor—we'll call him Father Mark—summoned Tom into his office. Where, he asked, was he thinking about applying to college. Boston University, Tom said. He wanted to go to B.U. A fine institution, Father Mark replied, though not a Jesuit one. Your father and I have talked it over, and you'll be attending Georgetown. One imagines Father Mark having this conversation again and again, throughout his career, with every graduating boy. At the end of the fall term, he made some calls. To Fathers Mike and Paul and James—admissions directors at various Jesuit schools, each of whom was told how many boys Father Mark would be sending him. No entrance exams, no admissions essays. After college came law school, after law school the partnership. A neatly plotted life, divergent in only one respect. He'd married, had a son, divorced. Nevertheless Tom remained an ardent Catholic, dismayed at the "permissiveness" of Vatican II, the masses in English, the focus on poverty.

They met through my father, who knew Tom from an insurance case he'd been assigned to investigate. The couples double-dated; during holidays, cookouts, birthday parties, Tom and his wife would stop by with their son, Ed, who was a year younger than Chipper. They were my parents' friends, adults, the wallpaper of childhood. My parents were the first to get divorced.

After my mother's divorce became final, after we moved to my grandparents' house, Tom began to visit. Red roses appeared by the dozen, fresh ones each week. For my mother there were dinners in restaurants with wine lists and candles. For Chipper trips into the city with Tom and Ed to see the Islanders or Mets. We were a cobbled together family, uneasy with each other, but to outsiders we must have passed—parents, two young boys crashing bumper cars into each other, scarfing down hot dogs, and playing Chuck Berry's "My Ding-A-Ling" on the diner jukebox, their older sister doing her best to ignore them all.

Unlike my father, Tom was steady, paid alimony and child support, kept appointments, indulged his son. My mother could be certain of him; certain, too, of her own appeal—taller, younger by nine years, a red-headed beauty with a sharp wit and an ability to get along, several steps up from the doughy first wife, who threatened to withhold visitation rights the few times Tom ran late returning their son to her home.

My mother and Tom were fixated on Watergate, though they interpreted it differently. For my mother it was all about hubris. She reveled in Nixon's downfall, said They should get him on Cambodia, too. Tom, on the other hand, thought Nixon had gotten a "bad rap." It was the media's fault. Them and the liberals who wanted to take everyone's money away and give it—plain out *give* it!—to the poor. A bunch of welfare cheats. People should pick themselves up by their bootstraps, that's what they should do. And what, my mother would ask faux-sweetly, what of those people who did not have boots?

We did not have boots. Or, rather, they were borrowed boots, ill fitting. When we moved to Tom's house, I got a new set of white enamel bedroom furniture, a stereo, a black and white TV. My brother, who'd been sleeping in the upstairs hallway, got his own room. There were vacations—to Nova Scotia, Lake Placid, to the lake house that belonged to Tom's brother, any place with water and fish. Through Tom's law firm we had box seats at Shea Stadium, ate in the clubhouse. Chipper saw Game Three of the 1973 World Series, attended the first game ever played at Giants' Stadium, saw Team Russia vs. the NHL All Stars at Madison Square Garden, where he rooted for the Russians because he knew it would annoy Tom. Lucky, his friends told him. You're so lucky.

As foreigners in someone else's home, we were made to feel the difference. Chipper and I were not spoken to, but were issued commands. *Clean Your Room! Stop That Racket. Pull Your Weight. Because I Said So. Straighten Up and Fly Right!*

Anything could enrage him. A sponge left in the sink. Toothpaste squeezed from the middle of the tube. The teacup I once ate ice cream from, instead of using a bowl. *TEACUPS ARE FOR TEA, GODDAMMIT!* Sputtering, red-faced, barely taller than Chipper, who was still years away from confronting him. My mother looked on, amazed. What the hell, she asked, is your problem?

Doors, cupboards would slam. The E-Z Listening station cranked up. A Beefeater's and tonic. And another, another. Yelling, *Goddammit, who touched the thermostat? You think money grows on trees?* Not every night, but often enough.

The thermostat, the dryer, hot water for the shower—all dangerous. Our jeans took longer than his polyester shirts to dry. When the half-hour timer went off, we were to hang them, still damp, over the shower rod, where they'd stiffen. Once when Chipper went over the half-hour limit, Tom presented him with the electric bill. My mother got her piggy bank, told us to get ours, too. We sat at the kitchen table, piling up change: pennies, nickels, dimes in columns. As we did this, we began to laugh, making a game of it, the absurdity too much, cheering when someone found a quarter, gasping with laughter, my mother's eyes wet. Tom sat in his chair, rattled his paper, muttered, finally slammed his way to bed. But he took the money and later threw a circuit in the fuse box to disable the dryer until my mother threatened to publicly shame him by doing laundry at the coin-op.

She lost patience. Couldn't we just go along with him? At least stay out of his way? We tried. Chipper made small talk about sports; I practiced avoidance. But we were teenagers. Chipper ate voraciously. I hogged the phone. We played our records loud, had poor table manners, forgot to turn out lights, rushed through chores. My mother placated, interceded. Some nights she lost her temper, matching him scream for scream, slam for slam. We hid in my room, knowing what was coming. *Kids, get your coats!* And we'd speed around town in my mother's VW, no one talking, nowhere to go.

Cheapskate, she called him, the worst of names. People had an obligation to share; she'd learned that from her mother. Even when money was tightest, during my mother's childhood, but especially once she had an income of her own, my grandmother was on the lookout for people with less. Widows she could invite home for the holidays, down-and-out families who needed a bag of groceries. She wasn't religious, never went to church. But childhood poverty had taught my grandmother empathy for the poor. Through a colleague she'd learn of some struggling family and "adopt" them for Christmas, enlisting her own family members in the effort: money from her grown daughters, toys from her son, a check from her husband. *A hundred, Jim, not fifty, we can afford it, don't be a cheapskate!*

Reluctantly, my grandfather went along. Poverty had taught him a different lesson altogether. Best to hoard, hard times could come again. Didn't she know that? Besides, look around—they weren't exactly living like kings. But no, she said. They had a home, a television, plenty to eat. Grown, healthy kids. A hundred dollars, what was that?

She loved to spend, but spent little on herself. Holidays she'd splurge, call Gold's Delicatessen weeks ahead of time. *Bernie, this is Mrs. McTigue. I have a big order; I hope you can handle it.* Tubs of coleslaw, potato salad, platters of roast beef, smoked turkey, paté with chopped egg, mounds of Kaiser rolls and special, brown, "holiday mustard." Papery slices of provolone and Swiss, pimento-stuffed olives, celery sticks with spreadable cheese. She mounded food until our paper plates sagged, too much food, all the food she'd gone without. She could give us, her grandchildren, things she'd been unable to give her daughters—trips to Dairy Queen, take out pizzas and lo mein. More than enough. *Eat! Eat!* The children in Africa. We heard about them, yes. Leftovers were sent to the "adopted" family, a post-Christmas meal. Who cared if she'd ordered too much? The important thing was to share.

My mother absorbed this lesson. She wrote checks to anti-poverty programs, became foster parent to a Native American girl, made us donate something each Christmas to the church's toy drive, an event Chipper and I agonized over because we knew if we selected anything too obviously neglected or worn, anything she knew we didn't at least somewhat care for, she'd override us and make the choice herself. Feeling the loss was part of the point. Besides, she said, you know you'll be getting more.

To my mother, Tom's wealth was a moral handicap, something that blinded him to other people's plights. She enjoyed that wealth—the trips to Florida, the dinners out—just as I liked having a TV and stereo. Yet his privilege pained her, the way it stunted him, the distinctions he made—who was worthy of largesse, who was not, how little it had to do with need.

Our own need had abated. Despite Tom's theatrics over bills, there was money to spare. We had allowances, three dollars a week in addition to lunch money. I bought nail polish in garish colors: watermelon, hubcap, pond scum. Chipper bought base-ball cards. We both bought albums. In exchange we were given chores. Chipper clipped metal rings from cases of tonic and 7UP bottles for recycling. He emptied the humidifier, trimmed rhododendrons, mowed the lawn. Winters he shoveled, falls he raked. He did this, as he did most things, cheerfully. It wasn't his nature to complain.

I was given lighter work. Vacuuming, dusting. I did these tasks on Saturday mornings while Tom slept so I could be back in my room before he woke up. I came down for dinner but would not speak. It wasn't the chores I minded; it was everything else. I sat at the table and burned.

My mother indulged my moodiness. We colluded. I hated going to school in my brace. One day a week she let me stay home provided my grades did not suffer. She'd tell Tom I had a doctor's appointment, study hall, the excuses varied, and that she'd drop me off on her way to work. I'd get up, dress, wait for him to leave.

On these hooky days, I mostly watched reruns. *F Troop, I Love Lucy, Twilight Zone, Bewitched,* the more fantastic the better. I'd lie on the couch, shoulder blades touching metal, close my eyes, and listen. Genies, time machines, talking mannequins, witch cotillions, there were lives in which anything could happen.

Whenever Tom took Chipper into the city for a game, my mother and I would get deli sandwiches. She'd pour me a small glass of wine, the sweet Almaden she and Tom drank at dinner. With no one to pound on the bathroom door, she'd let me out of the brace so I could take a long hot shower, water coursing down my itchy back.

Sometimes I was even excused from family outings. My mother's new sister-in-law had a house on a lake. Hers was a large, boisterous clan; they sailed and swam and skated. I could not lie on my towel in the sun, go in the water, balance on skates. Because of this, I was granted the luxury of staying home. I'd sleep late, my family gone to eat hot dogs and swim. Alone, I blasted the air-conditioner and stereo, ate cereal from a teacup, watched television, did laundry, running the dryer on high for as long as I wanted. I went into Chipper's room and my mother's, looked at the things

there: baseball books, pennants, bottles of perfume, tubes of lipstick in shades of rust and orange, Tom's pile of *Playboys* on the
floor by his side of the bed. I went through them. The women's
bodies—glossy, impossibly sculpted—made me feel slightly afraid.
Was this what one was supposed to become? I wanted my family
to come home and dreaded their return.

Orphans

Sometimes I feel like a motherless child
A long ways from home . . .

I hated those lyrics, one of the songs we sang each Sunday at St. Pius Church. Folk Mass took place in the All Purpose Room, a brick box that during weekdays served as the school cafeteria and gym. A room dense with massed bodies, candle smoke, embedded smells of cabbage and sweat. Instead of depicting gospel scenes, the windows were threaded with chicken wire. We sat in rows of folding chairs facing the altar, and the lyrics we sang were printed not in the leather bound missals I associated with church but in mimeographed booklets, crookedly stapled. These, I recall, had crude line drawings—doves, lambs, headstones. Chipper and I were not Catholic, had never been confirmed, but when my parents divorced, the high Episcopal church we'd been attending, with its incense and pomp, its ladies in white gloves and veiled hats, became for my mother an unwelcoming place. No longer a role model, she was relieved of Sunday School duties. *Perhaps you don't care for your children's spiritual development,* Father Matthew wrote when she was recuperating from surgery to repair a slipped disc. Some Christians! she scoffed. Has anyone bothered to see if we're okay? If maybe you kids need a ride? She crumpled up the letter.

In this new church, my aunt's church, we wore jeans and sang songs to end the war. A girl in bell-bottoms shook a tambourine, a longhaired boy strummed guitar. From his altar, a large table used for lunch time with a cloth draped over it and a cross set on top of that, Father Mike led us through "Where Have All the Flowers Gone?" At the time I was too young, ten or so, to be embarrassed by the treacly lyrics. The song, with its evocation of dead soldiers sprouting flowers from their graves, fit my budding pacifist sensibilities. I was a hippie wannabe, what I knew about hippies coming mostly from episodes of *The Mod Squad.* "Blowin' in the Wind," which we also sang, had lyrics as cryptic as the book titles in the adult library. I knew the lyrics by heart, sensed that the song was some sort of hippie anthem. But the motherless child song upset me. Instead of protest it offered up pitiful images of orphans. Singing it, I could see the Ghost of Christmas Present with that bone-raggedy boy, that jaundiced girl huddled beneath his robes: *This boy is Ignorance. This girl is Want. Beware them both, and all of their degree, but most of all beware this boy . . .* Children unloved and unloving, what had they to do with ending the war? I changed the lyrics to mimic a popular candy bar jingle: *Sometimes I feel like a nut. Sometimes I don't.* I mouthed these new lyrics to Chipper; we whispered them. To him it was funny, a way to get through the most boring hour of the week. For me though the song was deeply disturbing.

During my first summer in the brace, my mother decided to have her tubes tied. A routine procedure, she assured us, nothing to worry about, women did it all the time. She'd be home from the hospital in a couple of days.

I was not reassured. The last time my mother was hospitalized, for a slipped disc, our lives had been disrupted. My grandparents came to stay with us in their former home. Because of my grandfather's Parkinson's disease and, more to the point, my grandmother's "nerves," Chipper and I were forbidden to go outside. You'll fight, my grandmother said. Throw rocks at each other, fall out of trees and break your arms, get bit by a dog. Your grandfather's sick; I can't be running to the hospital all the time.

She ordered Chinese food, pizzas, took us to Dairy Queen. Manic from sugar and MSG, cooped up indoors, we fought. You kids! You kids! my grandmother wailed. You make me so nervous!

Rising from his La-Z-Boy, my grandfather would teeter on his way to the bathroom, grab at furniture, his feet shuffling wildly. He'd get stuck in doorways, something about the transition between rooms short-circuiting his already damaged nervous system. I knew he would fall but when he did, pitching forward, landing on his hands, the impact—his body hitting the floor, glassware rattling in the drain board, the needle skudding over vinyl, my grandmother's shriek, and the awful silence from the rest of us—made me want to hide.

My grandfather was dead weight, helpless. It took all of my grandmother's strength to help raise him. Jim for Chrissakes stay in your chair, she yelled. Everybody . . . you make me so GOD DAMNED NERVOUS!

My father's mother was called in. She took us on long drives, let us play shuffleboard at the seniors' home where she lived in a one-room efficiency. On my birthday we went to an Italian restaurant with my father, whom she'd persuaded to come along. He gave me a crushed velvet floppy hat and a string of love beads that I wore every day until they became unstrung.

That night I cried myself to sleep. It was my birthday, my tenth birthday, and I wanted my mother. I hadn't spoken to her since she'd left. Each time the phone rang, I was convinced it was the hospital calling with bad news. People told me she was doing fine. How was I to know? And if she wasn't, if they were lying? What then?

Nearly four years later, my mother was again in the hospital. I wanted to think myself stoic this time, able to cope. I was not the girl who wept at imagined funeral scenes, the girl afraid of the ringing phone. In truth I was even more anxious than before.

This time we stayed with Tom. Now was his chance to get back at us for all the times my mother had intervened. He could disable the dryer, make us wear wet clothes, take cold showers, scrub floors, haul trash; he could refuse to feed us, withhold our allowances, take away my stereo. None of this seemed to me far-fetched, but in fact he left us more or less alone. Unable to cook, he brought home Big Macs and boxes of Kentucky Fried Chicken. These were treats, but I could not enjoy them. Most of my plate went into the trash. Tom ate later, by himself, sandwiches or scrambled eggs. He might ask Chipper how his day had been or whether we'd done our chores but that was the extent of our interaction with him. We could shower or not, eat or not, wear clean clothes or dirty. So long as we kept quiet and stayed out of his way it didn't matter.

After dinner we went to my room. We played our music low. She'll be all right, won't she? Chipper would ask, and I kept saying yes, but secretly I had my doubts. With my mother gone, what was our connection to this man, this house? She'll be fine, I said, because the alternative was unthinkable, although I never stopped thinking it.

The day after my mother's surgery, Tom drove us to the hospital for a visit. Pale, perspiring, my mother lay on her back. It hurts, she moaned. It hurts so much. She looked at us briefly then shut her eyes. Her lips were chapped white, her bangs soaked. A bag hung from a metal pole, dripping fluid into a tube taped to the back of her hand. I tried not to look. A nurse came in, told us visiting hours were ending. We'd been there less than an hour. I knew we'd been brought to say goodbye. I'd read Dickens, knew what happened to orphans. Sure, there were no workhouses any more (were there?) but children without parents were still in for a rough time. I ran down the list of potential caretakers.

My father. Hopeless.

My grandparents, elderly, sick.

My uncle, just out of college.

My aunt with four children and another on the way.

It was possible, I reasoned, for Chipper to escape the orphanage. Tom might keep him. Someone to do yard work, watch ball games with. But who would want a moody, physically deformed teenaged girl? I was headed straight for a life of rags and gruel, a life where no one cared if I wore my brace or not, my spine growing more crooked until I was hunched and bitter, a fairy tale crone.

Perhaps this was already happening.

Because my mother was too weak to brace me, even after she came home, I had nearly a week of freedom. I could sunbathe, douse myself with the garden hose, wear a bathing suit, sleep unencumbered. I did all these things, enjoyed none of them. That is, I did them all with a sense of guilt. Drifting off to sleep I'd think, *I should be in my brace.* The only reason I wasn't had to do with my mother's fragility, which diluted whatever pleasure I may have, must have felt. No one else cared enough to restrain me, day after day, absorbing my rage. No one else held up the prospect of my future.

My mother was the sole capable adult in my life, the only one both willing and able to care for me. The brace served as physical reminder of my dependence on her. Without it, I was unmoored. Without it—without her—there was no telling what might happen.

She recovered, of course. My furlough ended. Once again I yelled, protested and scowled, all the while happy, secretly happy, that I was being forced to bear the thing I loathed. One reprieve had come to an end, but another more important one had been granted.

Monkey Girl

Stick up the butt. Tin Can. Hey, Robot! You sit like you got a broom-stick up your ass. So-and-so loves you; he wants to go out with you. Kissing noises, grunts. I ignored the boys' jeers. The girls were more polite; they left me alone.

Step on a crack, break your mother's back. A childhood refrain. Was my back broken? It needed propping up; I needed propping up. In the refrain, a broken back is the worst of maladies. We'd jump over cracks to avoid its curse.

Ten months before my birth, my mother's first child, a ten-month-old boy, had died of spinal meningitis. I knew this, knew there had been someone before me, the shadow of a baby, the mention of whom can still make my mother cry. Growing up, I rarely thought of him. I was the oldest, the first; I knew there had been someone else, but that was a long time ago, before I was even born.

You were in a glass bubble. I wouldn't let anyone but your father and grandparents hold you. My friends had to put on a hospital mask and gloves before I would let them into the nursery. I was terrified of germs, terrified of losing you. Thank goodness your brother was born and forced me to ease up.

Strong, athletic, easy in his body, Chipper was my physical opposite. As a child he could not sit still. My mother had a wire playpen installed in the backyard. When Chipper screamed to be let out, she would toss him cookies. Later she had a fence built, one with a locking gate. In third grade, Chipper's teacher tied him to his chair with jump rope and he ran around the room, chair strapped to his back, trying to make the other kids laugh. He played baseball, hockey, built forts, rode his bike into town to blow his allowance on candy. Playing Superman, he'd crashed through a screen door, splitting his lip on the concrete porch steps. Twice he'd cracked open his head. For fun he and his best friend held "dart wars," ducking for cover behind couches and chairs, lobbing darts at each other's head until, injured, Chipper ran crying to my mother, a dart stuck in his forehead. So rambunctious was he that once, in the crystal and glassware section of a department store, my mother's best friend grabbed him by the arm and said, Chipper Horvath, you behave yourself right now. We don't have time to go to the emergency room today!

Chipper never teased me about my awkwardness, my inability to ride and run and play sports. Perhaps he sensed this area was "off limits"; perhaps, given how inept I was, he just didn't see the point. Certainly he felt sorry for me, my restricted freedom, a point driven home to him each spring when my mother took him to the pediatrician for a scoliosis screening. One afternoon a year, instead of playing baseball, he had to bend and stretch while the doctor examined his spine. He complained. *This sucks; it sucks you have to do this all the time.* But empathy extended only so far in either direction. My love beads and hippie hair, the way I talked to myself yet clammed up in front of others, all of these were fair game as were his afro, his preppy clothes, his fear of the dark.

We posited ourselves as opposites, each having carved out a place in the family. The smart one vs. the athlete. The introvert vs. the friendly kid. The one you'd want to help with your homework vs. the one you'd want to hang out with. I was jealous of Chipper's prowess, his ability to make friends, and doubtless he was jealous of the easy A's I brought home while he made do with B's and C's. We fought, called each other names, even pummeled each other before I was braced. We were siblings; we could do that. Let anyone else make fun of me, though, and Chipper would intervene, standing up, saying Leave my sister alone! He was big, it always worked, the bully backing down without a fight. Chipper was like an older brother in that way. But he was two years younger than me and because of that age difference we were in separate schools the entire time I wore a brace.

In Home Ec, girls talked about their periods; they talked about boys and kissing. My period had not yet come. I was flat-chested, my "bras" like cut-off undershirts with lace for affectation.

We were becoming sexual. We wore flavored lip-gloss, nail polish. I grew my nails long, shellacked them with glitter. The fast girls wore mini-skirts, blue or green eye shadow. Everything about them ready. They kissed by the lockers, necks craned back. Cried in bathrooms, their friends in a circle, commiserating. Girls on the rag. Girls whispering in study hall, She's *so* on the rag, I'm on the rag, who has a Kotex? I started high school two months shy of my fourteenth birthday and still not on the rag.

I knew about periods, of course, knew what to expect. One afternoon in fifth grade the school nurse had shown the girls a movie—*Why Can't Jane Go Swimming?* or some such. It would be messy, we were told; it might hurt. Perhaps, for no clear reason, we would cry. The stories we'd been told about the Tooth Fairy, Easter Bunny, and Santa Claus had all been lies. There was no free money, candy, toys. Jesus on the cross however was real, and to prove it, each Sunday we'd dressed in scratchy clothes and knelt in pews where we heard sermons denouncing us as miserable sinners. From this I concluded an early, important lesson. If the story concerned suffering, it was likely true. If treats were promised, it was probably a lie. Menstruation was inevitable, only when?

The nurse had demonstrated a sanitary belt: a white rubber device with metal clasps dangling from it. The belt went around one's waist, and a thick sanitary pad attached somehow—I was not certain how—to the clasps. My mother had one of these belts on the top shelf of the linen closet. The pads were maybe half an inch thick—diapers for women. The apparatus had baffled me; for years I had shut it from my mind. But now I began to wonder how I'd

manage. Would the belt fit over my brace? How, without bending, could I attach the pads? Would the metal clasps click against
the corset, announcing me? No one had mentioned tampons; they
were not for "beginners." But if I had known about them (applica-
tors! strings!) I doubtless would have found them scary. I wanted
my period, wanted to prove that in at least one respect my body
was normal. Yet I was relieved when it didn't come.

In high school there were two other girls with Milwaukee braces.
One came from the junior high across town. Although we had
different schedules, we would pass each other in the hallways. As
strangers, we never greeted one another, never acknowledged our
shared disability. She had long blonde hair, a face that was pretty
and benign.

The other girl upset me. She was severely disabled, one
among a group of about twenty Down syndrome students who
had classes in the building. These students were notorious in our
school for the disruptions they caused. They raced down hallways,
knocked into people, stripped off their clothes, locked themselves
in bathroom stalls and would not come out. Once a Special Ed
student crammed a watering can's spout up the faucet then turned
on both taps, flooding the bathroom. Of course these students
were irresistible targets for the tough guys.

The Special Ed kids ate during Fourth Lunch shift, which
was also when the kids who took shop and auto mechanics ate.
It was the worst shift; people were hungry, the cafeteria ladies
were packing up, the pizza had run out. Fortunately, I only had
Fourth Lunch during math, every six or seven days on our rotating
schedule.

We had twenty-five minutes. The Special Ed kids clogged the
line. They screamed for cake, smeared mashed potatoes in each
other's hair; they dropped their trays and cried. Behind them, the
tough guys made bleating noises. They shouted. *Hurry up, retards.
Morons. Fuckin' geeks!* All during lunch the tough guys kept this

up. They lobbed milk at the Special Ed students' heads. They pitched pennies and laughed at the frenzy to retrieve them. No one ever told them to stop.

In English we were reading *Flowers for Algernon* in which the narrator, an intellectually disabled man, undergoes some kind of experimental therapy that slowly transforms him into a genius. He recalls how throughout his life people he'd considered his friends had mistreated him. Being in ninth grade, I took the theme to mean "Ignorance Is Bliss." But I didn't really believe that. The Down syndrome kids, with their food-matted hair, their foreshortened limbs and submerged, aquatic faces, were a source of derision. Not even their teachers protected them. To me their ignorance seemed something awful.

The tough guys singled out the girl in the brace. They called her the same names they called me, made the same kissing noises. Rather than feel sorry for this girl, I felt repulsed. My disability had made me watchful, even passive, a passivity I believed was sometimes mistaken for a lack of intelligence. After all, I'd been forced into sixth grade guidance sessions with the slow girls just because I wouldn't talk. Each semester on the Honor Roll was a triumph I was never entirely convinced I could repeat. My brain set me apart, just as my body did. Now I worried that people would conflate this girl's dual disabilities, somehow seeing them both in me. In some fundamental way the girl with Down syndrome threatened my sense of self. Every time I saw her, I quickly turned away.

Larry Doyle had been harassing me since sixth grade. I hated everything about him: his greasy Hitler hair, his crooked smirk, and his untucked flannel shirts. He made monkey noises at me in the hallway. I'd walk past, a monkey indeed, hear no evil.

Maybe it was that smirk. Or disgust at the way he and his friends threw pennies at the Special Ed kids. Or anything, nothing, I don't know. He was coming toward me. Making monkey noises. Before I could register what I was doing, I blocked his path.

He scratched his armpits and hooted. Fuck you! I yelled. People around us stared. Larry stared. I felt scared, exhilarated. What would he do? He couldn't hit me, he'd hurt his hand on the brace. I wanted him to do something so I could scream at him again.

To my amazement he snuck around the corner, shoulders hunched, eyes downcast. Neither he nor his friends ever bothered me after that. Had I finally shown them what they wanted to see? That I had feelings, I could crack? Or were they simply as scared and limited as I was?

Chastity Belt

He licks his index finger, touches the paper where it burns too fast. Passes me the joint. Slow, he says, take it slow. He leans in, cups his hands to my face.

New Year's Eve. Carol's brother Steve is teaching us to smoke pot in the woods behind their house. At first I choke, feel nothing. Steve pats my shoulder. Easy, he says. The joint goes around. One of Steve's friends sparks a new one.

So quiet in the woods, I can hear twigs fall. My jacket with the fake fur collar is too flimsy for winter, but I do not feel cold. The sky is vast, bright with stars. The archer, the crab—who saw such things in them? Why not the rock star, the giant cat, the chocolate bar? I begin thinking up my own constellations. The joint comes around. Someone laughs and says, Patti's stoned.

I'd made two friends, nondescript girls from chaotic families. Janine's parents fought incessantly, her Sicilian mother wailing— *Porca miseria, I've ruined my life!*—her father, screaming back in Yugoslavian, heaving their possessions into the street. Dishes, records, a bowling ball, even the vacuum cleaner. What an asshole, Janine would mutter as we cowered in her room. We listened to music for hours. We drank her father's homemade wine and watered down the dregs.

Carol's parents were rarely home. Professional cellists, they were away at performances, practice, tutoring jobs. She and her three brothers had the run of the place, so we spent most of our time there.

Hers was a house filled with boys—her brothers, their friends, cars in the driveway, music blasting, people stopping by, raiding the fridge. Steve was sixteen, shiny blonde and acned, the introvert in a highly social family. I liked him simply because he talked to me, asking questions about books I'd read, turning me on to new bands. But our relationship was platonic. I was the Girl in the Brace. I could never be his—or anyone's—girlfriend. He already had a girlfriend, a freshman like us, and he spent a lot of time at her house. When he was home, he or his friends would sometimes share their weed with us. These were boys with facial hair, cars, spending money. Voices that had broken and were disconcertingly low. Gentle, directionless boys who excelled at nothing in particular, who lived for music and pot. We did not know them, their parents, where they lived, how they acted in school. They appeared from nowhere, a boon. I felt shy around them.

We'd troop into the woods then sit around the den, my girlfriends sprawled on couches, me upright in a straight-backed chair. The pot made everyone quieter, introspective; it made me feel centered. The boys talked more than we did. Janine and Carol cast furtive glances, flipped their hair. Shaped their mouths into perfect O's when the joint came around. They began to wear midriffs, low cut shirts, dangly earrings. Janine sat leaning forward, her shirt hiking in back, revealing the perfect, knobby alignment of her spine.

At home, unshackled for my shower, I would run my hand along the planes of my torso—my bones as sharp and smooth, I imagined, as polished dominos. My hair was long and wavy. To make it longer I straightened it with a curling iron, let it curtain my face. Wiped steam from the medicine cabinet mirror, where I could not see below the neck. Pushed my hair aside and stared at my reflection. I practiced the expressions I'd seen my friends make—The Pout, The Arched Brow, The Alluring Smile. I was not beautiful, but I could pass for pretty. How was anyone to know?

I spent my days in bedrooms—my own or the bedrooms of friends. We stacked albums in milk crates, kept a steady rotation on the turntable, painted our nails, played with make-up we'd swiped from Caldor's, lounged around like odalisques, me sitting on the bed, rigid. Sometimes they went to the beach, its heat and shimmer too much for me, all those glistening bodies. I'd spent days there as a child, digging in the sand with Chipper, eating gritty hot dogs and candy necklaces, but now I preferred the movies. It didn't matter what. For a few daylight hours I could linger in air-conditioned darkness, the theatre nearly empty, row after row of balding velour seats.

Summer nights I went outside. We'd sit on Carol's front steps flicking ashes onto the cement, smoking down to the filter, flipping butts into the bushes. I didn't like cigarettes, didn't even inhale, but the gesture felt purposeful. We spent whole evenings like this.

Couples formed. A hand on someone's knee staking a claim. An arm around a waist. Not my knee or waist. Boys would stop by Carol's house and stay even when Steve wasn't home. They offered us rides, night trips to the beach. I tagged along. I was for safety, a chaperone for girls who did not want to go too far, at least not right away. A couple in front, one in back; me, unable to bend, leaning back at a forty-five degree angle next to some boy, not my boy, close enough to smell the tobacco on his skin, the soap traces in his hair, his sweet pot breath. Summers the tidal reek came in all briny; winters the windows fogged. After we'd done a few hits, the driver would start the car. I'd be home by nine.

Saturday nights my mother and Tom went out. I'd heat frozen dinners and watch the television line-up: *Mary Tyler Moore, Bob Newhart, Carol Burnett*, the room loud with canned laughter. Chipper would eat a bowl of ice cream then go to bed at eleven so he could be up for hockey practice by five.

The romances of fourteen-year-old girls are brief. No one wanted to go all the way. Everyone wanted to look around. There were so many boys. After a break up, my friends were briefly disconsolate. They'd call me up and cry. I was the sympathetic ear for their sagas, the metal shoulder to lean upon. Eventually, though, they would relax back into themselves, talking a little louder, asking if I wanted to go hang out at Caldor's, complaining that, once again, there was nothing to do.

Percentages

This fifteen-year-old girl has a four-year history of idiopathic scoliosis. She has been treated for a two-year period with a Milwaukee brace. Despite the use of the brace, she has had a mild progression of her curve and is admitted for a spinal fusion. At the time of admission, the patient had a right thoracic and left lumbar curve . . . x-rays show a curve to the right from T-6 to T-11 of 45 degrees, and to the left from T-11 to L-5 of 49 degrees. . . .

— *Dr. Wayne Southwick, Chief Orthopedic Surgeon*
  Yale New Haven Hospital

The School of Medicine, Section of Orthopedic Surgery, Yale-New Haven Hospital, was far nicer than the Bridgeport clinic, with magazines in the surgeon's waiting area, an actual room as opposed to a hallway, one with carpeting, end tables, freestanding chairs. To me, these details were unsettling. They emitted a visual warning: You have entered a formidable place, do not be lulled into comfort.

Even without these cues, I knew that this appointment was different, more serious, than any of my previous ones at the Bridgeport clinic. Dr. Wayne Southwick, whom we were scheduled to see, was a renowned orthopedic surgeon, "tops in his field," Dr. Mangieri had said. Getting an appointment wasn't easy, both for insurance reasons and because of Dr. Southwick's schedule. My mother recalls that Dr. Mangieri had first needed to make a presentation, detailing to a number of other physicians, Dr.

Southwick among them, the history of my case. This presentation had taken place at the Bridgeport clinic. I have no memory of that event whatsoever, yet my mother insists that I was there.

The presentation was so clinical and cold. It was like you were a specimen, as though you weren't even in the room. You weren't a patient, you weren't a young teenage girl, you were "the case" with "the deformity." I thought, Oh, my God, this is so hard to hear. I just wanted to scream at him: "Shut up, don't say these things in front of her—she's human!"

A nurse showed us to Dr. Southwick's office, where I changed into the hospital gown, tying it as tightly as I could. I shivered, not just from the cold November day or the flimsy gown, but from all that a hospital gown entails—vulnerability, the transformation from person to patient, the ceding of self. The office was spacious and light, so different from Bridgeport, with a large polished desk, family photos, and a nautical theme dominated by pictures and sculptures of whales. I hoisted myself onto the examining table. My mother sat in a small chair. To while away our long afternoons at the Bridgeport clinic, she'd taken up needlepoint and was working now on a complicated piece depicting a fire-breathing Chinese dragon. If we spoke about anything, it was mundane. I was too frightened, I know, to focus on what might come next.

Soon a tall, white-haired man entered the room and, nervous, I stood up from the table. He walked over to us, shook first my mother's hand then mine. Even from a distance of thirty years I can recall how he spoke to me directly, using language a teenager could understand. I was more than a body gone awry, he seemed to say; I was a person, someone about to endure a lengthy ordeal. It was important that I understand what he needed to do and why.

Dr. Southwick explained that the spine is the supporting column for the entire body. Mine was twisted from mid-spine to base, unable to do its job. A mild curvature was considered to be less than thirty degrees; severe curvatures were greater than sixty degrees. I fell somewhere in between, a bit closer to "severe" than "mild," but the brace clearly wasn't working. Without surgery, Dr.

Southwick continued, I could become stooped, my lungs compressed, weighing on my heart, damaging it. Breathing could become difficult; there was risk of long-term pain, pneumonia, even a shortened lifespan.

I had just turned fifteen and was still growing—crookedly. The time for surgery was now.

Calmly and with great precision, Dr. Southwick spoke to me, his words revealing my future. Two metal rods, one to support each curve, would hold my spine in place and keep the curvature from worsening. My vertebrae would be fused from mid-spine to base with bone grafted from my hip. The operation would take five or six hours, and I would remain in the hospital for about three weeks. At first I would be in a plaster "shell," a kind of holding cast for my torso. A week or so after surgery, once I had sufficiently healed, I would be set into a chin-to-hip plaster cast. This cast would extend to the knee on one leg; I could choose which leg. I would spend three months in this cast, flat on my back, able to move both arms and bend one leg, unable to sit up, raise my head, roll over.

After three months, I would be cut free and placed into a lightweight fiberglass cast. I would have to relearn how to walk. My spine, Dr. Southwick explained, would be permanently fused, unable to bend. If all went well, he could remove the fiberglass cast in another four months, after which I would begin to gradually wean myself from the brace. The entire procedure would take about a year.

All of the springs and straps, the rashes, lesions, and sleepless nights had not sufficed to keep my spine in place. Now we would use steel rods, implanted in my body. I tried not to dwell on the details, the girl on the table, anesthetized, swaddled in plaster, immobile. *Step on a crack and you break your mother's back.*

Three or four times we made the trip to New Haven to consult with Dr. Southwick. The hospital was almost an hour away, and on these days I did not go to school. After each visit, my mother would take me to lunch at the Rathskeller, a nearby German restaurant that I liked because it was wood-panelled and dark, full of Yale students, people whose age I could imagine being. They laughed and were loud and confident-seeming in their bodies. I'd order a Reuben, and my mother would let me have one of the dark beers that arrived all frothy in a cold-beaded stein. On the drive home, feeling drowsy, I'd shut my eyes and sleep. The next day was a school day, one more in an endless stream that would eventually lead to my life.

I resisted surgery in a way I had not resisted bracing. The thought of being helpless terrified me. Sentenced to bed for months, able to use only my arms, unable to bathe, feed myself, use the bathroom—I told my mother I would gladly forgo surgery in exchange for a few years at the end of my life. My father's mother was stooped, yet she drove and painted and played shuffleboard and no one had fused her spine. I resented my mother, my brother, their big compliant bodies, my mother's ability to press her palms flat to the floor, Chipper's baseball mitt, hockey stick, football helmet, and bike.

I threatened to run away. My father lived in Manhattan; occasionally Chipper and I visited him for weekends of Chinese food and HBO movies. I harbored fantasies of moving in, knowing he was far too negligent to ever concern himself with my health. I'd sleep on the pullout couch, stay up late, never wear my brace or go to school.

I proposed alternative treatments. Chiropractors could straighten spines. Acupuncture—why not? A girl at school told me about a faith healer who had sent someone's cancer into remission. Crackpots, Tom said. This was not medicine—sanctified, insured. My mother had been told my condition was life-threatening, and that was that. We would get a second opinion, but only from another surgeon.

Late in the year we drove to Hartford, to the Newington Children's Hospital, formerly the "Hospital for Crippled Children." The waiting area, with its stuffed animals and children's magazines, exuded a feeling of clinical well-being, if not actual safety. I was hopeful. Nothing this doctor told me could be worse than what I had learned at Yale; logic dictated it must be better. He would take a wait and see attitude, counsel patience, more exercise. I'd bring up chiropracty and he would stroke his chin and say *Hmmm . . . yes . . . let's discuss that.*

Instead he told us, quite brusquely, that surgery was in order. He recommended a longer convalescent period in a shorter cast, but the details were more or less the same. He had, he assured us, done many such operations and had never botched a single one. Of course spinal surgery was extremely complicated. Even a slight mistake could result in the patient's paralysis. If, however, he were to paralyze me—and there was a two percent chance of this—*I would hang up my shingle for good.*

My mother stared him down. I knew that look. In all the years of dealing with orthopedic doctors, therapists, x-ray technicians, receptionists, insurance companies, of driving to strange and seedy places, waiting for hours, absorbing my anger and fears, she had never lost her composure, but I could tell she was on the edge, her lips pressed together, her eyes small. Curtly, she thanked the doctor and told me we were leaving—*Now!*

All the way home I cried. The doctor's words had not been a balm. Fewer than five percent of adolescent women have scoliosis, a statistic I had learned. Of those, most do not require bracing. Of those who do, I had been told that ninety percent respond favorably to treatment. I was already a percentage of a percentage. If I underwent surgery, why wouldn't I be paralyzed?

This time we did not stop for lunch. My mother gripped the steering wheel so hard her knuckles turned white. Arrogant bastard! she muttered.

My mother spent the weeks before my surgery on the phone—arranging for tutors, time off from work, insurance coverage for a day nurse, a rented hospital bed. She brought out the sewing machine and made bed jackets: a reversible quilted one, red and blue, a floral cotton short robe; she splurged on a sheer white jacket with bell sleeves from Bloomingdale's. These were all I would wear for the next three months.

Tom wisely did not engage me in conversation, but he no longer complained about my loud music, my bad table manners, and my general hostility. Chipper lent me albums and even offered to let me borrow his portable eight-track player. But he was always nice to everyone, even Tom, even when he was being yelled at for running the dryer or leaving on a light. What I wanted was someone to share my anger. I felt duped. For three years I had had the false solace of believing my condition temporary. I would exercise until my back grew strong enough to change the course of my spine. I would wear a brace until I stopped growing. I would have surgery, but eventually walk again, unencumbered. Now a new possibility had arisen—I would be crippled. I would never drive, dance, swim, have sex, marry, no one would want me. Chipper would move out and I'd be stuck living with my mother and her miserable husband until they died and then . . . what? Thinking this, I could make myself cry, and crying felt good.

In Hospital

I could walk and then I could not.

I walked into the hospital; three weeks later I was wheeled out on a stretcher, loaded into an ambulance, and driven home. Between these two events, there is much I do not remember. For nearly a week I was sedated on morphine. My recollection of the days immediately following my surgery is sporadic, deeply synesthetic. Clammy blue hospital slipper socks, odors of ammonia and overcooked vegetables, bursts of flowers—carnations, roses, lilies—their browned petals spilling onto the windowsill in the overheated room. Wheezing from the bed across the aisle, a bed around which the curtains remained steadfastly closed. This raspy sound was all I heard late at night when the adolescent ward, so noisy during the day, was distilled to eerie silence and my need for morphine had wakened me again. For narrative details I rely on my mother, who understandably does not wish to dwell here. Already she had lost one child, her first, to sudden, inexplicable disease. The next one was about to undergo potentially crippling surgery. I can't begin to imagine the anger and helplessness she must have felt. When asked about it, she pushes at the air, pushing that time back into the past where she wishes it would remain.

Just before your surgery, I was lying in bed one morning and I felt I would never be able to get up. I felt this tremendous weight on my chest—real weight, not symbolic. I thought, I can't do this, I can't make her suffer any more. You were so scared. Remember that sonofabitch doctor who told us you might be crippled and how he'd stop practicing if that ever happened? All he cared about was his reputation. And I thought how can I make her go through with this? But here were these doctors—experts—saying we had to operate. So I just lay there, angry at everything—at God, fate, the universe—whatever had put you in this situation. And I didn't know what to do.

Then a thought came to me, out of nowhere. All you can really do is show your kids how to live with adversity. That was it. That's what I had to do. Deal with it and get you through. And the weight lifted.

In telling me this, she begins to cry. Why do you want to know? she asks. Why go back there? It's a good question. Writing, especially memoirs, is a perverse inclination. All of that dredging up of unpleasant memories. Implicating others in one's own narrative. Why go back indeed? Yet the past refuses to remain in its neat little coffin; one may as well push at air. Our histories haunt us. I am still the Girl in the Brace, still relearning how to walk. Though no longer visibly disabled, my self-perception has been irremediably altered by my experiences.

For thirty years I did not speak of this. Like my mother, I wished to bury the past. Bone disease changed that—forcing me to confront my own complicity in my decay. Let loose from my cage at age seventeen, I began to starve myself. It was not difficult to do. I had coffee for breakfast, spent my lunch money on yogurt and weed. We were a household of two working adults and two teenagers. My mother worked longer hours once my recuperation was complete, woke at dawn on Sundays to drive Chipper to hockey practice, ran errands for her bedridden mother who called several times a day demanding booze, cigarettes, ice cream, emphysema medicine. She enrolled in night courses at the local university. Meals were on the fly, and sometimes my mother did not have time to eat. Rather than have us sit at the table with Tom, who didn't want our company in any event, she permitted Chipper and me to eat on TV trays in the den. I picked at my food, filled up on salad, said I'd had a big lunch.

I wanted, I think, to punish the body that had caused me so much trouble. Doubtless vanity figured as well. For three years I'd been encased in metal, plaster and fiberglass. I'd been poked at, prodded, ridiculed, ignored, had suffered insomnia, welts, heat rashes, and for nearly four months I'd been unable to move. Set free, I wanted to physically break with my past, to be noticed for the shape I imposed upon my body rather than the other way around. At 5' 8" and 103 pounds, I was the thinnest girl in the room. Meanwhile my bones, starved of nutrients, were beginning their slow erosion.

I try to explain this to my mother. I tell her I've always seen myself as two selves—functional mind, dysfunctional body—one to be cultivated, the other endured. It is a self-conception that still holds. Yet by internalizing this identity—the disabled person who is no longer seen as such from outside—have I not caused myself harm? My inability to synthesize these selves, the privileging of mind over body, caused me to shun food, physical activity, and the outdoors long after my cast came off. I've even adopted a motto—"You're always better off indoors"—that I use whenever some well meaning person (invariably male) suggests a hike in the woods, a jog through the park or, worst of all, a camping trip. The great craggy vistas of the American West do not inspire me, except as landscape to be imbibed discretely and at a remove— in the photos, say, of Ansel Adams or Lee Friedlander. I see their cacti, their plains and buttes, and no lyric strain of rugged individualism swells my heart. I feel no desire to hike the lonesome trail, pitch my tent beneath the stars, sing odes to the lonesome prairie. A walk around the Harlem Meer will do just fine. My friends attribute this antipathy to bookishness. But it's more complicated than that. I've never learned to fully inhabit my body, to see myself as physically capable. My grappling with the past is more than a desire to piece together events; it is an attempt to forge an integrated self. To do this, I need to ask questions.

For one entire day I did not have to wear my brace. I checked into the hospital the day before my surgery for preparatory x-rays and lab work. Between appointments, I wore jeans and a turtleneck, luxuriating in the softness of my clothes against my skin. That evening a nurse shaved me front and back. When she left I splayed my fingers against my stomach, still pink from the razor. I twisted in front of the bathroom mirror to glimpse my unscarred back. I showered, changed into my pajamas—no hospital gown! no brace!—and thought I am doing these things, I am brushing my teeth. The other girl in the room was, I'd been told, "a bad case." She moaned and wheezed and her parents did not speak to anyone. They sat all day behind the curtain that encircled her bed. No one said to me, *See how much worse*, for which I was glad. It was not a comforting thought.

Just before Lights Out I was given a sedative and another in the morning before the orderlies put me on the gurney and wheeled me to the operating room where, surrounded by strangers, I was alone. Beneath his green surgical cap and mask I recognized Dr. Southwick. He said good morning; he said relax. The anesthesiologist hooked me up to an IV. He said count backward from one hundred, and I began.

Patient was brought to the operating room, placed under general anesthesia, and intubated. She was then turned in to the prone position on rolled towels and the back was prepped and draped in the usual fashion. A straight longitudinal incision was made from T10 down to the sacrum. . . . The first Harrington rod was placed from a sacral bar to L2 on the left side. The Harrington rod, the second, was placed from L4 up to T10 on the right side. . . . A large amount of cortical bone was then obtained from the right iliac crest through the same incision. . . . Prior to the placement of the bone graft, all wounds were debrided with a water-pik. The graft was laid down with care to place most of the graft on the concave side of all curves. . . . Hemovacs were inserted prior to closure. The wound was dressed.

The patient was placed in a posterior plaster shell. She was then turned into the supine position, extubated, and was sent to the Recovery Room in satisfactory condition.

—Dr. Wayne Southwick, Chief Orthopedic Surgeon
Yale New Haven Hospital

I do not know how long after surgery I regained consciousness, how much time elapsed before I again took note of my surroundings. The surgery took over six hours. Throughout that time, my mother and my father's mother kept vigil. They sat together in my hospital room, my grandmother moving her lips in silent prayer, my mother embroidering a whale for Dr. Southwick's office—a propitiatory gesture, appeasing fate via the almighty surgeon. They took turns at the pay phone, brought each other coffee, did not eat. Still doped up on anesthesia, I was wheeled into the Recovery Room, an event I do not recall.

From my mother's college English paper:
The first thing Pat said after surgery was "I can wiggle my toes, I'm not paralyzed." She thought she might be paralyzed because one of the many doctors we consulted before deciding on surgery kindly volunteered statistics to this teenage girl, citing the chance she would have of walking away from surgery. He remarked that if he ever paralyzed anyone he would hang up his shingle. We weren't interested in his ego-trip, our concern was the impact of this news on an adolescent who knew she already fell into the ten percent of scoliosis patients who did not respond satisfactorily to bracing and therefore faced surgery or the risk of shortening her lifespan. The possibility of becoming a victim of another set of statistics terrified Pat.

Fluorescent light sharp in my eyes, a dull sheen of bed rails, petals the color of blood, everything too bright. A pain in my bladder where the tube was stuck. My grandmother's veiny hand. Someone moaning, bovine, not me. Curtains being drawn around my bed, cloistering me.

It hurt to pee, it hurt to breathe. My urine came in crystals, and the catheter would not be removed until I could "make a stream." There was the problem of my lungs. They needed air. A tube was inserted down my throat; the other end attached to a machine that forced cool steam into my lungs. *In Out In Out—Good!* The nurse kept chanting. Each breath a slicing of my lungs. I tried to move my arms, I tried to pull out the tube. Gently, the nurse took hold of my right hand. My left hand, the one I wrote with, was taped to an IV. The machine pumped its steam, forcing my lungs to work. I took tiny breaths. My mother smoothed my hair and murmured words of soothing.

Between shots of morphine I slept, waking to ask what day it was when mere hours had elapsed. Gradually I became more aware of my pain, more aware of how little I could move, not even my arms, though I had been told I was not paralyzed. My body was in shock and needed to recover. Soon enough I would be able to raise my voice, and I did—for blankets, for socks, for morphine—mostly for morphine. After an injection I would drift as though wrapped in some warm fleecy cloud, floating above where I lay motionless. I had no body then. Slowly the heaviness would return, the pain. By the final hour I was dry-mouthed, fixated on my shot. I watched the clock. The hands would not budge. Five minutes then five minutes more—this stretched out for years. A buzzer looped around the bed rail, just within reach, but it was pointless to ring it before the appointed time. I rang anyway. I sweated, groaned, tore at my cuticles, drawing blood. I rang and rang. I felt every inch of my ravaged spine. Often by the time the nurse arrived I was in tears. The injection swept that away. Its effect was an immediate sweet languor.

My veins began to collapse. Bruises formed on both my arms. One morning a technician came to change my IV. He had trouble raising a vein. The rubber tourniquet pinched my arm as he tapped here and there, searching for a spot. *They're so small.* He complained, angry at the difficulty I was causing him. By now I could move my arms and I folded them against my chest. He pried them apart. *There! Got one!* He jabbed me, the needle jiggling in my vein, sending fire up my arm. I let out a cry. He tugged at the needle. Already a lump was swelling where he had missed, a tiny loaf rising in my forearm. *Other arm.* Again he missed, the needle dangling. I felt as though my veins were being scraped clean. *Too small, I can't get a good one. We'll try the feet.*

I was terrified of what this needle man might do next. I begged him to go away. He untucked the covers, exposing my feet. He told me to stop being a baby. Hysterical, I began to cry. The needle man readied his needle. I screamed—NO—and my mother came running into the room. She'd just arrived, still wrapped against the cold.

Don't let him touch my feet! I wailed. He's hurting me!

She pushed the technician away from my bed. I could not stop crying. My mother stood between my bed and the technician. She ordered him from the room, then found the head nurse who found someone from pediatrics, adept at locating a baby's sliver of vein. From then on a pediatric technician administered all my injections, and the bruising subsided.

The nurses were harried; they did their best. Each day they washed me, brushed my teeth and hair, gave me liquids, then Jell-O, then solid food. This meant I needed a bedpan, a new humiliation, and the nurses did not always arrive on time. I drenched my sheets more than once, developed rashes. For over an hour I was left on a fetid pan until my mother showed up. Told how long I'd been waiting, she threw a fit, the only time I heard her raise her voice at anyone involved in my care. Her frustration, like mine, encompassed so much more than this single act of neglect. It was boundless and had nowhere to go.

Postoperatively, the patient did well. Her wounds healed primarily. On the second postoperative day, the Hemovacs which were inserted at the time of surgery were removed and the patient transfused appropriately for her postoperative blood loss. By the tenth postoperative day, the patient's wounds had healed sufficiently that it was possible to remove the sutures and place her in a localizer cast with the right leg included.

*—Dr. Wayne Southwick, Chief Orthopedic Surgeon
Yale New Haven Hospital*

My painkillers were switched from morphine to codeine, from injections to pills. I no longer needed an IV drip. I ate hospital food: fruit cocktail, pudding, runny meatloaf, limp vegetables. Dr. Southwick judged it time to set me into the cast.

Ten days after my surgery, a gurney was wheeled into my room and raised to the level of my bed. Only a nurse and an intern were available to move me and because I was still in a temporary plaster "shell," my spine fragile, it was important that I not be jostled. The nurse asked my mother to help lift me from the bed to the gurney. Worried that she might drop me, my mother refused. Get another nurse, she insisted, get someone else to help. The ward nurse dismissed our fear: We don't need to get someone else; it's all right. But it wasn't all right and my mother wouldn't let them move me until another trained person had been found to help.

I was taken to a large, well lit room where Dr. Southwick waited along with several others: nurses, interns, technicians. My memory of the event is hazy. I was given a sedative and laid face up on a high table. First the plaster shell was severed along the sides and the top half pulled from my body. I was rolled over, face down, and the other half of the shell was removed, leaving me exposed. The gauze I'd been wrapped in was snipped away. I could feel scissors, cold on my skin. Dr. Southwick examined the scar that ran, I knew, from the middle of my back to my tailbone. The others crowded in to compliment his work, remarking on how fine the incision was, how pencil thin, a masterwork.

I may have been x-rayed, I don't recall. My impression is that Dr. Southwick oversaw the procedure, but did not actually do the work himself. From chin to hip I was wrapped in gauzy cloth like a kind of body stocking. A nurse held my head. Someone asked which leg. Being left-handed, and stronger on that side, I chose my right leg, which was then wrapped to the knee. Plaster soaked bandages were laid on my back and sides while I lay face down on the table. At first the wet plaster felt cool, almost refreshing, but gradually it heated up. Layer after layer was smoothed onto my back, neck, and thigh. I could not see anything, but could hear the slap of bandages, feel them hardening to a crust. When the last layer dried I was rolled onto my back and the procedure was repeated. Leg, hips, stomach, chin, bit by bit I was entombed. The bright lights the technicians needed to work by made me sweat inside the plaster. Another nurse wiped my forehead. *Just a little longer, that's it, good girl, we're almost done.* This went on for hours. When they finally finished, I was too heavy to be lifted but was rolled, with great effort, back onto the gurney and into my bed where I immediately fell asleep.

It wasn't until the next day that I realized how small my new world had become. I could bend one leg and move my arms. My neck was cemented in place. I could see nothing but the ceiling. In order to read I had to hold a book above my head, which made my arms tire. I could not see the person standing by my bed unless I rolled onto my side, but the cast was too heavy for that. My skin was sticky and hot. For the next three months this chrysalis was to be my home and I the pale naked larvae waiting inside.

I recalled the story of Giles Corey, whom we'd learned of in eighth grade English while studying the Salem witch trials. Accused of being a warlock, he'd been crushed with stones at the age of eighty-three. *More weight*, he'd cried when pressed to repent. *More weight.* I thought about his lungs, organs and heart yielding. I wanted morphine. Instead I took the codeine I was offered, thinking that if I stayed drugged enough, I could maybe sleep my way through the next three months.

Without the ability to turn over, I could not feed myself. The shell had left both my legs free, but now my range of motion was impossibly small. Each day a physical therapist worked with me on "mobility." I gripped the bed's metal guardrail and practiced heaving myself onto my left side, easier than my right, where the leg cast made turning difficult. Nurses slipped pillows under my head to elevate it slightly, and in this manner, lying on my left side, I practiced using a fork with my right hand. I hadn't anticipated this, the awkwardness of eating right-handed when I was a lefty, the way the leg cast would prevent me from lying on my right side. At first food went everywhere. Discouraged, I stuck to liquids taken through a bendable straw. To entice me into eating, my mother brought me pizzas, deli sandwiches, chocolate cake. The nurses, deflecting my frustration, joked about how much better my food was than hospital food. Patti, one nurse cracked after I'd spilled another plateful of food into my bed, I swear your middle name is make-a-mess!

The therapist showed my mother how to move me so that I would not get bedsores, how to slide a bedpan in and out, how to wrap plastic around the cast when giving me a sponge bath, how to wash my hair with a bucket and shampoo board. *Lift her head like this. Roll her this way . . .* I was constantly being pushed, tugged, rolled this way and that, the body in the bed, useless and inert. During that first week in the hospital, my mother was a near constant presence on the adolescent ward. She knew the nurses by name, when their shifts changed, who was quick with a bedpan or shot, who needed prompting. She brought them candy; they let her stay past visiting hours. Because her visits were long (and because he was thirteen and hyperactive and, I found out much later, afraid) she did not bring Chipper. My mother and grandmother were my daily companions, but I had other visitors as well.

My aunt came with chocolates and cards my young cousins had crayoned. Carol and Janine came for a visit during which Janine nearly fainted. A nurse had come to tend the other girl in the room, the "bad case," and had left the bed curtains open. The girl was groaning. Janine glanced over. I could not turn my head to see, I don't know what she saw. Suddenly she blanched and grabbed the bed rail. She sat down, head between her knees. The nurse asked if she should bring a wheelchair but Janine refused, frightened I think of being mistaken for a patient. It was easy to be frightened when one never knew precisely what to expect.

For patients, there was the uncertainty that accompanied our surrender to care. Visitors experienced the anxiety and helplessness of seeing a loved one suffer—seeing, by extension, themselves. Perhaps it wasn't the other girl who made Janine react after all. Perhaps it was me. The patient is a powerful mirror. There's nothing like a hospital to make someone, even a teenager, aware of mortality. The visitor thinks, There but for the grace of God, yet knows that this is false. There but for the time being. The relief of walking away, through the revolving doors and into the cold night air, comes as a shock. Years later, visiting a friend with AIDS, I would go straight from hospital to restaurant, to binge on sushi and martinis.

The Conversation Issue arose. How to talk to someone laid up in bed for months? What to say? Not even that old standby the weather was any help. One afternoon my father arrived with a pastrami sandwich he'd bought for me in New York. I suspect my grandmother had badgered him; nothing but her words could convince my father to set foot in a hospital. He was a man who took his temperature incessantly whenever he caught cold. A man who called cancer "the Big C" and menstruation "that female thing." Someone who had waited in the car whenever my mother needed to buy Kotex. Probably he'd been hoping to find other visitors in my room, but on this afternoon I was alone. My father's discomfort was palpable. He did not know where to look. He waved the sandwich, a trophy, and asked to sign my cast. "To a great kid!" he wrote on my torso, adding the word DAD in giant block letters. I think that's when he noticed the second gold stud in my left ear, a fifteenth birthday present from my mother. Piercing, he decreed, was barbaric. I reminded him that he liked boxing. That was different, that was sport. I did not know what to say about sport. Two healthy men pummeling each other's bodies. The visit was brief and my father did not return.

My cast took up some of the conversational slack, becoming a slate on which visitors could convert their unease into pithy slogans: "Hang in there!" and "To a great kid!" People drew flowers, cats, butterflies, geometric designs with bright Flair pens. Will you keep the cast when it comes off? I was asked more than once. The idea horrified me.

Cards, flowers, gifts piled up on my bedside table and windowsill. My mother's friends sent necklaces and earrings I could not wear. Their cards said I was "brave," a word I rejected as false. I felt helpless, far from brave. I no longer did things, but things were done to and for me. That word, "brave," mocked my enforced passivity.

Of course what could people say? Our language for illness and disability is so paltry, we often conflate them. "How long will you be sick?" I was asked. "I'm not sick," I'd answer testily. "I'm in a cast." Sickness was unpredictable, dangerous. In the hospital, the distinction was especially important. Sick people did not go home.

Lights Out

When the "bad case" was moved from my room to critical care, I was not sorry to see her go. More than anything, I wanted to escape. Sedatives allowed this, but my sedatives had been diluted from morphine to codeine to Valium, a near placebo. The other girl's noises had kept me awake, trapped inside myself. I'd stare out the window at the New Haven city lights and listen to my roommate dying, believing she could not hear me, even had I been able to summon a word or two of comfort.

The nurses moved in a new girl, someone who spent her days in the patients' lounge, where kids without visible ailments sat in their bathrobes, watching TV. I no longer recall what she was in for, but she seemed blasé about her time in the hospital, which turned out to be brief.

This new girl was a fireplug who swore and chewed gum and shared the pizza her parents brought. After Lights Out we'd stay up late talking, her bed curtains open. I began to feel less alone. One afternoon, toward the end of my hospital stay, Denise brought a boy into our room. She explained that she'd met him in the lounge and had told him about her roommate who could not move. He'd wanted to meet me.

Yes, I thought, yes, come see. The girl who cannot move. One look and you feel better about yourself, don't you? I didn't say that. I wanted to turn from him, this boy whom Denise called Jimmy, this boy who wanted to see. But I could not.

So, he asked, what happened?

Dummy, my roommate responded, I told you, she has a fucked up spine.

He asked how long I had to stay like that. Denise said she didn't know. Not forever? he asked and I said around three months because I was tired of them talking about me over my head. Three months, the boy said, that sucks. You should get out of this room.

I looked at him then. A short boy, shorter than me, I suspected. Hunch-shouldered, with shaggy black hair that touched the wire rims of his glasses. An affectation of cool in a tartan plaid robe. He smiled. Did I want to get out of here? Go for a ride?

Already he was pushing my bed from the wall. I said what are you doing, we can't and he said why not and then we were at the door, Denise looking up and down the corridor, waving us on. I was going somewhere with a boy I'd just met but I wasn't afraid. The change of air, so slight, felt good on my face. We raced past the nurses at their station, past doctors and patients, orderlies with gurneys, grim-faced visitors, this boy, this stranger, taking corners, running down halls. I felt exhilarated—someone was finally making something happen.

He offered to take us to the roof and I said it would be too cold, which was probably true, but secretly I was concerned about getting in trouble, about being trapped with this boy. And yet, not. Part of me wanted to say, Yes, let's escape, anywhere not here. He wheeled us back to the adolescent ward where a nurse asked what we thought we were doing. Just going to the lounge, he said, and she said, Make certain that's all.

We watched television with the other kids until it was time for dinner. After the trays were cleared, Jimmy came to my room. He was evasive about why he'd been hospitalized, saying only that he had "stomach problems" and would be operated on in the morning. When I asked what was wrong with his stomach he said he didn't know, probably the hospital food, which, I agreed, sucked. But why was he eating if he was having stomach surgery?

You ask a lot of questions, he said.

We talked about music, school, our families. He was a freshman, half a year younger than me. His father was a judge, his mother stayed at home, he and his brothers, all older, went to private school in a town more than an hour from where I lived. The summer before he'd hitchhiked to Florida; I'd never been anywhere alone. He'd had girlfriends, knew all about drugs, could get me, he boasted, whatever I wanted though I did not yet know, aside from pot, what precisely that meant. We held hands, something I'd never done. Denise returned, complaining that there was nothing on TV. A nurse announced Lights Out and Jimmy kissed my cheek.

Denise sat by my bed, talking about Jimmy. He liked me, did I know that, did I know he didn't have a girlfriend? Too bad he was leaving in two days. Two days? My stomach lurched in its plaster casing. Surely she was mistaken. He was having surgery, needed time to recover. But that's what he'd told her, she was sure. Already I was missing him, feeling sorry for myself and wondering at that. Denise kept talking . . . *you can always phone, it's not like he's in Alaska or something, maybe he'll come visit and . . .* We heard a scuffling in the hallway, slippers on linoleum. Jimmy ran into the room. He wanted to say good night, he wasn't sleepy, who the hell went to bed at nine, what the fuck?

The night nurse had a way of announcing herself, a horsey gait. Jimmy ducked into my closet. Denise ran to her bed. The nurse flipped on the light. Denise yawned and stretched, pretending to be awakened from a deep sleep. I put my hand over my mouth.

The nurse was looking for someone. We knew who, she knew we did, and if he was found in our room . . . well, he better not be, did we understand? Perhaps she suspected he was hiding and chose not to look. What could happen? Jimmy did not stay long. He kissed me chastely on the cheek, slowly kissing his way toward my mouth, small pecks, moving closer. Good night, he said between kisses. Good night and good night and good night. He took off his glasses. I shut my eyes. I wasn't certain what to do. I let him, he seemed to know, and then I was kissing, all broken and hot.

My sense of hospital time is attenuated. Looking back, it seems Jimmy and I were together in the hospital for weeks, but this cannot be. He was there for only a couple of days. I next saw him in the afternoon, miraculously recovered from surgery, which, he confided, was actually a circumcision, not a stomach operation. He mumbled as he said this; he looked at the floor. I said something to the effect that all boys have those—don't they?—only why, I wondered, did his parents wait so long? He didn't know. He offered to wheel my bed around the ward again, but I did not want to see anyone else. When my mother came to visit, she found us alone in my room holding hands. I pulled my hand away, stuck it under the covers. Jimmy stood up, shook my mother's hand, introduced himself. The hunch in his shoulders disappeared. He seemed confident, as though he'd spent a lot of time talking to girls' parents. My mother gave me the "Who's this?" look. Had I been able, I would have shrugged. I did not think I would see him again, so I did not think it mattered.

That night he promised to visit me at home. He'd hitchhike, he said, take the train, what was wrong, didn't I believe him? Of course I did, I told him so; I believed he meant it. I also believed he'd forget all about me the moment he went home.

In the morning he came to say goodbye. He wore jeans, an untucked oxford shirt. His mother was waiting, he could not stay. Already he belonged to that other world, the one where busy people moved about freely. He kissed me quickly, turned to leave, came back. I wanted to hold him, get out of bed, hug him goodbye. I opened my arms. It was all I could do. Jimmy put his knee on the mattress. He leaned over me. I reached up and pulled him against my body cast. I could feel his shoulder blades, the muscles in his back. I wanted to remember him. His hair was coarse. His body felt small and strong. My body was concealed. There was only my face, which he kissed—nose, cheeks, mouth. I have to go, he said.

All the Difference

I was sedated for the ambulance ride home. I do not remember it—the shock of February air, whether the day was sunny or dim, nor if the orderlies chatted with me. Did they blare the siren? Was my mother in the ambulance?

I went to the nurses' station to order an ambulance, my mother said. And they told me, Oh, you don't need an ambulance, just borrow a station wagon and put her in the back. Like maybe you were the groceries. You realize she can't move, I said. You realize she's in a hospital bed and can't sit up. They got the ambulance. I made sure you were strapped in safe and then drove home and the ambulance followed.

I was carried on a stretcher into the house, through the living room and up the stairs. I have a vague recollection of dizziness, of seeing familiar objects from unfamiliar angles. My mother had rented a hospital bed and I was settled there beneath a mound of blankets and the pink and green spread that my father's mother had crocheted.

An adjustable hospital table had been set up beside my bed. It became a catchall for books, paper, pens, tissues, water pitcher and glass, telephone, hand mirror, brass bell. The telephone was a private line that my mother had installed while I was in the hospital. Like my bedroom walls, comforter and sheets, it was pink, a pink Princess Trimline with a push button dial in the receiver. The dial lit up so I could make phone calls in the dark, late at night, when I was supposed to be sleeping.

With my hand mirror I could see the outside world, reflected through the window behind my bed. By tilting the mirror just so,

I was able to glimpse my mother's light blue Volkswagen, Tom's dark blue Audi, two or three bare-boned trees, a snowy patch of yard. In this way, I watched the days change. The bell belonged to my mother's mother. Its brass was etched in a swirling pattern, and the handle was teak. Before my surgery it had been displayed on a three-tiered mahogany shelf, part of a motley collection of treasures that included two powdered geisha dolls in red silk kimonos, a floral porcelain demitasse set, a Royal Doulton clown mug and a brass opium pipe. I had needed permission to touch any of these things. Now I rang the bell, a princess, whenever I needed food, water, a bedpan.

For the bell to be heard throughout the house, my bedroom door had to stay open whenever I was alone. My sense of privacy was thus further eroded. Only at night, when my mother could hear me through our shared bedroom wall, was the door kept closed. Under the circumstances, I believe she had little difficulty convincing Tom to relinquish their bedroom stereo for the duration, enabling me to use headphones, the same headphones he'd ripped from the jack whenever I listened to music downstairs. Now they protected him from having to hear Aerosmith, Blue Oyster Cult, and David Bowie.

The stereo was relocated bedside, to a white enamel table. On its twin was a milk crate full of records. With practice, I learned to propel myself onto my left side, flip one-armed through the crate for the album I wanted, set it on the turntable, and hit the play switch. This proved useful the morning one of my caretakers fell asleep. I woke, needing the bedpan. I rang and rang the bell. I telephoned the other line. My mother would not have left me alone; someone had to be somewhere. I shouted—no use. Finally, despairing, about to soil myself, I had an idea. I put Led Zeppelin on the turntable, cranked up the volume on "Black Dog." It worked. The college girl my mother had hired for morning duty had fallen asleep on the couch in the den, two flights down. When she heard the music, she thought at first that angels were announcing some end of world event. Then she'd realized where she was.

I listened to records, watched TV. My mother had replaced my black and white set with the remote controlled television from her room, balanced high on the bookcase so I could see it from bed. Late at night, unable to sleep, I'd stay up watching whatever was on: reruns of *The Burns and Allen Show, You Bet Your Life*, or, if I was lucky, an old movie on *The Late Late Show*. I watched Marilyn shimmy in and out of trouble; Fred and Ginger, so liquid, glide through high society. Something about the night, its extreme stillness, discomfited me. If nothing was on, I'd read. But reading, my greatest pleasure, had a new way of exaggerating my sense of confinement. Because I could not lift my head, I could not read in comfort. I'd stretch my arms above my head until they ached then turn onto my side, which eventually made me cross-eyed. Then back again, lying flat, my arms tiring more easily with each attempt until, after less than an hour, I'd be forced to give up. Sometimes, edgy from a day of doing nothing, I implored my mother for Valium. Try, she would say. Try to sleep. Eventually she would relent and I knew this, knew the delay was a necessary ritual, her way of expressing concern that I might become addicted to the sedatives the doctor had prescribed.

Around dawn, with the first light, something loosened in me. I felt then that I could relax. Soon there would be noises in the house: water running, my brother getting ready for school, my mother frying bacon, voices in the kitchen. I would drift off, waking in the late morning, groggy, hungry, needing to pee, not always remembering what day it was and who would answer the bell.

During my second week in the hospital my mother had returned to work. This was economically necessary, but necessary too for mental health—mine as well as hers. She recognized that we both needed a break from her near constant care. My father's mother had been a nurse. She knew how to change a bedpan, give a shot, ward off bedsores. She came to see me often, and I knew she'd offered to help, but she was in her seventies and no longer capable of the hard physical work that caring for me entailed. My mother came up with a plan. She posted a notice at the local university for a part-time companion and aide. Five mornings a week, from nine to noon, one of three Fairfield University students stayed with me. MJ—small, blonde, perky—laughed a lot and made fun of herself. She was the one who'd fallen asleep on the couch. Sandy was dark-haired, stately, and tall. I thought her beautiful and was always a little startled whenever someone mentioned the wine-colored birthmark on her cheek because after a couple of days I stopped noticing it. Eileen, a nursing student, was serious and gentle. She tucked Saran Wrap into the openings of my cast and bathed me with a warm cloth. I'd kept my hair defiantly long, not cutting it for surgery, clinging to my pre-op self. Had I been able to stand, it would have fallen to my waist. Alone among the three of them Eileen brushed and washed my hair, sliding a shampoo board beneath my head, pouring heated water from a watering can, sudsing my scalp with manicured nails, my hair streaming into a blue plastic basin, the room fragrant with shampoo.

Very quickly I came to love these girls. They were like sisters, imagined ones, who never argued or fought.

All three whiled their mornings away in my room. They rolled me in and out of bed jackets, made breakfast, brought me orange juice, gossiped about their boyfriends, told family stories, complained about exams. But each weekday, promptly at noon, they were replaced by Mrs. Brattle, Visiting Nurse. This was a stringy woman in her sixties in full white regalia: clunky shoes, stockings, pressed uniform, starched white hair, and cap. Just seeing her made me feel like an invalid. Mrs. Brattle's manner was all brisk condescension and when I did not need her, she stayed downstairs. On her first day, she complained to my mother about my music. I knew this because my mother complained to me—about Mrs. Brattle. *A teenager, what the hell does she expect—Mozart?*

My mother called the agency. Someone younger, she said, someone who'd be good with a teenage girl. A shortage, she was told, we'll see what we can do.

I began treating Mrs. Brattle as I did Tom—someone to be borne, better ignored. When I needed the bedpan, I tried holding back until my mother came home. The university girls always laughed off my embarrassment, and I felt at ease with them. Mrs. Brattle fed me, wiped me, changed my sheets, but neither one of us deigned to speak beyond what was essential. Sometimes, when I couldn't sleep, I wondered about Mrs. Brattle. Did she have a family? Was there a Mr. Brattle? Did she like to read, watch old movies on TV? I never found out. She was there for business, and I was her job.

There were seven channels: three network, one public, three local. Weekdays the choices were soap operas (network), children's TV (public), or sitcom reruns, interrupted by long commercials for a host of strange inventions—a vacuum cleaner attachment that could be used to dry hair, mechanical knitting needles, a tool that transformed beer bottles into jewelry. I watched, knowing all the sitcom plots: the greedy would be punished (*Twilight Zone*), the bumbling rewarded (*F Troop*); the powerful woman (*Bewitched, I Dream of Jeannie*) would be humbled, but not before showing up her hapless, bossy spouse. I should have been doing homework, I knew, preparing for the tutors who would come after school. But I had scant interest in quadratic equations, igneous rocks, irregular Spanish verbs. I'd do the minimum required, just enough to get by, knowing my tutors would go easy on me.

Four hours a day I was tutored in each of four subjects: English (Mr. Martin), Geometry (Mrs. Rector), Earth Science (Mr. Dillon), and Spanish (Mrs. Kendall). I especially liked Mrs. Kendall, a grandmotherly woman, easily distracted. Whenever we approached the subjunctive, I would begin an exaggerated series of yawns, stretching my arms, making a cavern of my mouth. You must be getting tired, dear, she'd say. Let's try something else. And once again we'd go over the novel we were reading—about (I think) a saintly widow who was being either delighted or tormented (I was confused on this point) by her dead husband's ghost.

When I got bored with the woman and the ghost, I'd ask about Mrs. Kendall's granddaughter. Out would come the wallet snapshots: *There's Rosie's first birthday party. Look at her little hat. Oh, and she did the cutest thing with the cake . . .*

Late winter sunlight streamed into the room. Mrs. Kendall went on and on, her voice like water over rocks—soothing, soporific, expecting nothing in the way of real attention. After she left, I always napped.

I liked Mr. Dillon, too. He reminded me of Captain Kangaroo, if Captain Kangaroo had worn aviator glasses and carried around a bag of rocks. Igneous, sedimentary, metamorphic. Rocks born of fire, water, evolution, dull unchanging rocks taking shape from the earth's upheavals. I held them, examined their veins and glassy surfaces, this little bit of nature relocated to my hot pink bedroom. Mr. Dillon projected slides onto the ceiling—volcanoes, crashing waves. *The Origins of Earth.* He talked about rocks the way my friends and I talked about rock bands—reviewing their histories, their individual merits, playing favorites. I tried to share his enthusiasm; clearly the rocks meant so much to him. Is this really sedimentary? I'd say, picking up an igneous rock. No, no, he'd say again, patiently. Look at the veins! I could rarely make it through the two hours. Despite myself, feeling sorry for Mr. Dillon because he was trying so hard, my mind wandered. I nodded during slide shows, mistook stalactites for stalagmites, plopped Paleolithic rocks into the Mesozoic era. Okay, Mr. Dillon would say, defeated once again by my ignorance. Let's wrap up. Doubtless he was relieved at the prospect of early release from the bedroom of a bored fifteen-year-old girl.

Unfortunately, nothing could distract Mrs. Rector from her protractor and compass. Neither snow nor rain nor my vaudeville yawns . . . she was stolid, a post office of a woman, squarely built, every hair sprayed into place. Math was my worst subject. Mrs.

Rector and I slogged through equation after equation. She drew triangles, circles, trapezoids. We measured angles and curves and subtracted little y's from little x's. It was nearly enough to make me long for Mrs. Brattle.

Don't you think that's a bit adult for you?

I was reading *Catch-22*. It wasn't on the syllabus, but I liked it far better than *A Separate Peace*, which Mr. Martin had assigned. A couple of spoiled rich boys in prep school—what did they have to complain about? So Phineas was on crutches, so what?

Do you understand it? Mr. Martin asked.

I narrowed my eyes. Who did he think he was talking to? One of the cheerleaders whose flirtations made him blush to the roots of his scant blonde hair? A jock who needed vocabulary words explained because she was too lazy to look them up?

It's better than *Separate Peace*, I said. All Gene does is sit around and brood. Who cares?

I could, of course, have been talking about myself.

We read about Silas Marner with his miser's sacks of gold. We read Shakespeare's sonnets and Robert Frost:

Two roads diverged in a wood, and I—
I took the one less traveled by,
And that has made all the difference.

What difference? I thought. And what difference could there possibly be when others did all the choosing—what things would be within my reach, whether there would be water to quench, food to sustain, pills to soothe, whether curtains would be open or drawn, sheets rumpled or tucked, pillows flat or plumped, whether, indeed, I would be able to walk a road, any road, ever.

I could not walk, but I could talk; that indeed made a difference. Whether my needs were to be met, though, or when, or how, was up to someone else. The man who chose the road had no wrong decision to make. The fact that he could choose was enough and I resented his blithe freedom, my condition coloring all that I took in.

After the tutors left came the dead time of late afternoon—lessons finished, my mother not yet home, Mrs. Brattle busying herself somewhere in the house, out of sight but within earshot of my bell. Strangely, I have little memory of Chipper. Where was he during this time?

I was scared of you. I didn't know how to talk to you, what to say, so I stayed in my room a lot, hiding from Tom, listening to Kiss. Because it's your sister, someone you grew up with and fought with and still love, and she's in this iron lung thing. I was a little freaked out.

As he tells me this, I note the shift in pronouns, the direct address slipping into third person, "you" becoming "she." Even at a distance of thirty years, the visibly disabled must be kept at some remove.

He knows, he says, he should have been more present. I tell him it was long ago, he was thirteen and couldn't help how he felt; besides, a lot of people, much older people, were uncomfortable around me. Mrs. Brattle was paid to care for me, yet she barely came to my room. My father stayed away. My uncle sent Tolkien books. My aunt had five children to raise, and my maternal grandmother had her own difficulties just getting out of bed. None of these people, however, mattered to me the way my mother and Chipper did. None of them felt vital to my daily life.

Disabled people freak people out, my brother confesses. He's right, of course. I couldn't even look at the Down syndrome girl in the brace. Her dual disability—one so foreign, the other so familiar—freaked me out. And she wasn't even someone whose name I knew. I had no stake in her fate. It cost me nothing to avoid her, nor was she aware of my aversion. How much more difficult for a child to confront a sibling's deformity, the word doctors used to describe my condition. How much more painful for that sibling—the patient—to be shunned. Because we'd always been close, Chipper could not bear to see me, his anguish isolating us from each other, making of me a pariah.

As soon as she came home from work, before changing clothes or talking to anyone else, my mother would run upstairs. I'd hear her coming and a great feeling of relief would overtake me—someone to talk to, albeit briefly, a change in the tempo of the day. Later I would hear her making dinner, smell meat cooking. I ate alone. I did not want to be seen eating. When I needed something, I rang the bell. I rang for the bedpan, a new pitcher of water. I rang for pillows to be moved so I might try again to read. Chipper stopped in to say good night, sometimes carrying the cat, who fidgeted in his arms. I watched TV and rang for pills and eventually was given them so that I could sleep, waking once again to ring the bell.

Waiting

I have to hang up. I'm falling asleep.
Okay. Good night, honey.
Good night.
Honey.
It's four a.m.
Say it.
We've been talking five hours. I'm tired.
Say it. Let me hear you.
Good night . . . honey.
Good night. I'll call you tomorrow.

It was him on the phone, his voice. Late at night, a day or two after I came home. *I told you I'd call, didn't you believe me?* Waiting until his parents had gone to bed, and on those nights when the phone rang at eleven I did not beg for Valium.

What did we talk about? Who can recall? Music and school. Friends. His day, not mine. The parties he'd been to, the classes he'd cut. The calls went on for hours. Neither one of us wanted to hang up. I'd fall asleep to his voice: *Good night, honey. Say it, call me honey.* With the receiver pressed to my ear I listened to him breathing, a companion in the dark.

He told me, that first call, he was coming to see me. Friday, after school let out. He wanted to phone my mother, make certain he'd be welcome, and arrange a ride from the station. I didn't like this idea, thought it overly formal. I'd tell her myself. But Jimmy insisted, saying it was better for him to speak to my mother directly.

I told him when to call, a time when Tom would be at work. Make sure you talk to my mother, I said. Her husband's an asshole; he'll say no.

I knew my mother would be fine with Jimmy visiting, but I wanted to warn her about his call. I thought she might tease me, gently mock his propriety. Instead she seemed pleased, no doubt happy for the distraction. He has good manners, she said.

Friday evening she rolled me into my favorite bed jacket, the white one with sheer, belled sleeves. While she drove to the station, I brushed my hair to a high gloss. Sprayed my wrists with cologne—a hospital gift—Charlie or Bonne Belle. I never wore cologne, didn't like it, thought this was something I was supposed to do. Smeared on mascara, lip gloss. Someone, a boy, was traveling over an hour to spend the weekend with me—a girl who could barely move. I had to beguile, even—especially—if I didn't have the slightest idea how.

My mother's VW crunched into the driveway. I picked up the hand mirror, saw Jimmy, reflected, emerge from the car, saw him and my mother, tiny in the mirror, walking together toward the door. Suddenly I wanted to stop it, stop them, wind the reel backward. This was a mistake. I didn't know this boy, what he expected. Face to face we'd run out of things to say. He was on the stairs, in the hallway, knocking on my door. I swallowed, said come in. The shock of him, immediately familiar, that face I had conjured, goofy grin and floppy black hair. He'd brought gifts—a box of cheeses, a bottle of André pink champagne. He set them on the desk, hung his leather jacket over my chair. Smiling, easy, as though he did this every day. He looked at me, said my name. We were kissing like that. Then he pulled away.

What *is* that shit? he said, You stink, wipe it off! He brought me a warm cloth and I scrubbed at my wrists. Your face too, he said. Why are you wearing that?

And, as I washed away make up, cologne, I began to feel at ease. Here was someone who liked me without lipstick or manufactured smells, without ever having seen me from the neck down. It felt ridiculous, too good to be true, and I knew it was. But I felt something happening in that room. A kind of reverse transformation had taken place—the swan turning back into her duckling self—amazed that she should be met with approval.

We put records on the turntable, kissed through song after song. He opened a window, lit a joint, fanned away my exhaled smoke. We watched it dissipate. Ate cheeses from the cheese box—a waxed block of cheddar, a walnut-studded ball of orange cheese in crinkly red cellophane. Jimmy went downstairs for crackers and plastic cups. He didn't let me ring the bell, said let me do that, let me get things for you. We drank the champagne, fizzy in my nose, a sour candy. Before this I'd only had it on special occasions. This was a special occasion. Jimmy took off his glasses, dark hair falling into his eyes. He slept beside me, fully clothed, and we woke, our breath rancid with cheese, kissed some more, fell back to sleep. The weekend passed like that. We watched *Saturday Night Live, Don Kirshner's Rock Concert*. Friends stopped by and for once I wished that they would leave, as they'd wanted me to on those summer nights with boys, wishing I would leave so they could be alone, wishing I would linger so they wouldn't have to go all the way.

We couldn't go all the way.

We kissed, our lips chafing, shared a tube of cherry ChapStick. He changed in the bathroom. I had a face, arms. We lay together in the hospital bed, smoking weed. Jimmy stubbed the roach on my torso, an affront not against my body but against the barrier between us. He rubbed its mottled surface and I imagined I could feel his hand on my stomach, miles below.

Nothing made sense. Not just Jimmy, but me, in this bed, this cast, unable to move. There was my body, this failure, this wreck. There was this boy. How did they fit together?

Sunday was dismal, from afternoon on. I kept the time in mind, counted down the hours, then the minutes. He would leave, come back—the choice was all his. Jimmy hesitated saying goodbye, said *I have to go*, didn't. My mother knocked on the door. I waited for him to call, and he did, that night, and the next, and I understood that this was what it would be like between us—him coming, going, saying when, me waiting.

Tom complained. *She's on the God damned phone all night, I can't sleep.* I could hear him snoring, knew he slept fine. We communicated through my exasperated mother. *So she's on the phone, so what, how the hell would you like it, stuck in your room like that?* I knew I would win, but agreed to keep my voice down. I whispered through the night to Jimmy, the lighted phone dial glowing in the dark.

Phineas died; Gene felt guilty. We moved on to Julius Caesar.
    Volcanoes cooled to ash, this was igneous.
    The woman in the Spanish novel explained how she knew the ghost was her husband.
    $a^2 + b^2$ equaled c^2 and I did not understand any of it.

We were working on triangles. Right, acute, isosceles. All night I'd been talking to Jimmy. My eyes hurt; I couldn't concentrate. Mrs. Rector droned on. School had been called off for snow, but nothing could stay Mrs. Rector from her appointed rounds. I heard the front door shut—Chipper?—heard a commotion of voices: Mrs. Brattle's and, improbably, Jimmy's. I strained to listen. It *was* him, arguing with Mrs. Brattle, telling her never mind, he was going upstairs anyway. She yelled for him to stop. Mrs. Rector looked up from her book. Who was this boy, flushed with cold, snowflakes in his hair?

I hitchhiked, he said.

Nurse-busy, flustered, Mrs. Brattle burst into my room, demanding that Jimmy leave at once. Mrs. Rector cleared her throat. We had triangles to draw. Jimmy said he was going to shovel the driveway. Mrs. Brattle wrung her hands. *When your mother finds out.*

While Mrs. Brattle fussed and Mrs. Rector droned, while I seethed over the injustice of math lessons on a snow day, Jimmy shoveled the drive. He kept at it, even after Mrs. Rector left. I watched him in my hand mirror, wishing he would stop, wishing the sun would go down. Chipper came home. My sister's boy-friend, he told Mrs. Brattle. My mother knows.

Jimmy returned, smelling of snow, the outdoors, changing the air in my room. He shut the door. This was too much for Mrs. Brattle. Back into my room she stormed, followed by Chipper, who said It's okay, my mother lets her. There we were, three teenagers against a nurse. We'll see, Mrs. Brattle said. We'll see about that. Jimmy said, Shut the door on your way out. Chipper gave him a look. We could hear Mrs. Brattle on the phone. *A boy!* Her voice rose in agitation. *No one said anything about a boy!* But she left us alone after that.

My mother let him stay for dinner, after which she made him call his parents, who told him to come home. I cried and vowed never to forgive her. In the morning she phoned the nursing agency and said send someone else, I don't care who.

He brought me Cold Duck, pink champagne, a ceramic heart on a gold chain, a brooch in the shape of a turtle: *Like you.* He brought me *Frampton Comes Alive* and we made out to "Baby, I Love Your Way" and the long song with the wa wa machine.

We went nowhere, did nothing, stayed in bed, fell asleep while the TV turned to snow. He opened windows, letting in the metallic winter air. I clutched at the pink and green afghan and he pushed it aside.

Between visits he carved my initials in his forearm with a Swiss army knife, block letters that left rusty welts, his own scar—visible, self-inflicted, nothing like mine. When we've been together longer, he said, I'll do your whole name.

Late at night he told me all the things we would do. Hitchhike to Florida. Take the train to New York and visit his friends. Go to parties all night long. *When that thing comes off and I see what you look like—I bet you're so beautiful, I bet you're so fuckin' thin.*

He came and went. I waited. I rarely called because I didn't want to speak to his parents or brothers, to have to explain who I was, *that* girl, stuck in bed, all those towns away. Sometimes he would call from a party. I could hear music in the background. And girls, their high, bright, laughing voices. Girls I hated. Quit it, I'm on the phone! he'd say to someone I couldn't see. Hold on! Listen, I gotta go. I'll call you later.

I didn't ask when, though I always wanted to.

The new nurse looked like a child playing at being a nurse. Twenty-five, barely older than the college girls who cared for me, Betsy was pale, freckled, petite, with tiny hands. Even her voice was girl-ish, helium-tinged.

She wore her auburn hair pulled tightly behind her nurse's cap. Our first afternoon together Betsy asked about that cap. Did she really have to wear it? It felt so, well, formal. Goofy, even. I was delighted. You don't have to wear the uniform, I said, no one else around here does. Betsy asked my mother, who said, Call me Maureen. From then on she wore jeans to work.

I told Betsy I had a boyfriend who stayed with me in my room. It was a test.

She said she and her boyfriend, Frank, lived together; they were talking about getting married. When I could walk again she'd have me over for dinner. He was, she said, an excellent cook.

When the tutors left, in the late afternoon, Betsy would sit with me. She gossiped about the other patients she'd cared for—cranky old people who made her wear the uniform, cap and all; a woman who'd wanted her to do housework. Not the routine clean-up-after-yourself stuff my mother expected, but real housework: vacuuming, toilet scrubbing, dusting. She told me about her dates with Frank: dinners, movies, concerts, and I superimposed images of me and Jimmy, holding hands at the movies or sharing a meal at a small round table lit with candles, draped with checkered cloth. I had no knowledge of such a place; my restaurant experience was limited to Howard Johnson's, Pizza Pan, and Beefsteak Charlie's. Someone played "Bella Notte." We were Lady and the Tramp. We toasted, clicking glasses. I wore a low cut dress, dangly earrings, maybe a string of pearls. No one knew what I had been.

I lived vicariously through Jimmy and Betsy. After she saw Paul McCartney and Wings at Madison Square Garden, Betsy described the show. As she talked I thought about wings—not the band but the object: archangel wings, spiky and white; the waxy feathers of Icarus; a dragon fly's tapered, iridescent sheen, a butterfly's papery spread. I wanted wings. Betsy went on: the lines of white limos, the scalpers charging hundreds—*hundreds!*—of dollars for a single pair of tickets. The lasers and dry ice, how Linda McCartney stood robotic at her keyboards, the way the strobes beamed through a haze of pot smoke. So much smoke she'd gotten a contact high. And then *that* conversation: *Do you? Yes, me too.*

Don't tell. Not even Chipper.

She brought me some weed in a film canister, spread its contents onto a double album, using her driver's license to separate seed from shake, letting the seeds roll into the album's seam as I had done when I'd been able to sit up.

We were girlfriends. We were patient and nurse. She rolled joints, painted my toenails, rubbed lotion into my feet, made me bend my left leg so it wouldn't atrophy. She stood on tiptoe to change the sheets, faster than anyone, rolling me from side to side, whisking away the soiled set, tucking in corners.

My scar was healing and had begun to itch. Betsy devised a way for me to scratch with a chopstick, inserting it through the armholes of the cast. We ate the food she brought from McDonald's, listened to records from her collection, made fun of Tom, the awkward way he flirted with her, his cluelessness, his scuzzy polyester suits.

She got along well with my mother, put up with Tom, watched TV with Chipper while I napped. But she was mine, there for me. Chipper had his sports; my mother and Tom had each other. All of them had responsibilities to the world beyond my bedroom. Betsy did not, at least not during the hours we spent together. As the weeks went by, I began to feel increasingly dependent upon her—dependent and possessive.

The calls became less frequent. Shorter. He couldn't make it every weekend, no, of course not. There was school. His parents objected.

I tried to think of things to say. Stories to tell, ways to regale. I could move my arms. I could hold him.

I couldn't hold him.

Weekends became a trial. Friends stopped by, no different, really, from what we'd always done, hanging around, waiting for something, usually nothing. But then there had been at least the hope of distraction. Someone might call, someone's mother might offer to drop us at Caldor's or McDonald's; at worst, we could walk to the Bridgeport Motor Inn, steal change from the vending machines while the desk clerk watched TV in some back room, then spend the money next door at the Green Comet Diner on hamburgers and juke box songs. Something might happen; I could pretend. Now there was no pretending.

Jimmy came, took some Quaaludes, slept nearly the entire weekend. I was angry and the following weekend he didn't show up. Call someone, he said during another visit, one of those girlfriends of yours.

My body felt heavy, sluggish. I was becoming slow. It took me longer and longer to read a book. I'd reread sentences, lose my train of thought. Maybe it was the drugs. I was convinced I was becoming stupid, my brain atrophying in tandem with all my other muscles. Eventually I would become an oyster or jellyfish.

Through my mirror I watched snow melt, crocuses bloom from mud, brown grass turn green, the world in transformation. Branches grew fat with buds, the air warmed and mellowed. Betsy opened my window and I could smell the ripeness of everything. I hadn't felt the sun in nearly two months, nor the rain, nor seen beyond the world framed by my window. Neighbor kids shrieked at their games. I examined my face, made it slack. Two eyes, a nose and mouth. That was all. I ended at the neck. Who could love that, even believing it temporary?

We were on school break. The tutors stayed away. Jimmy hitched down, early afternoon. I was excited for Betsy to meet him. He hadn't visited in a couple of weeks, and I was hoping he could spend the night. But he showed up with a friend—a surly-looking kid, solidly built, a buffer.

Jimmy had weed. Colombian Gold, he said, holding up a baggie of yellow clumps. He rolled a fat one in bright pink paper. Strong, he said, hold it in. I did, keeping the smoke in my lungs for as long as I could. Betsy took a hit, said Good stuff. The familiar floaty feeling washed over me, a narcotic balm. Directly behind it, though, came a new sensation—my first experience with pot-induced paranoia. The music sounded distant, tinny, people's voices faraway. Jimmy was watching me; so was his friend. What did they see? I was sweating inside my cast, my skin trapped, unable to breathe. I could feel each damaged vertebrae. The cast bore down on me. I would never walk, never leave this room. Slowly I felt myself slipping away from my body, hovering somewhere inches above it, looking down at myself in bed. The room was saturated with color, a shimmer at the edges of things. I don't remember what I said, but Betsy began talking me down. She sponged cool water on my head, held my hand. It's okay, she soothed, everything's all right.

Jimmy and his friend left the room. When they came back I felt a little better, though still frightened. They whispered together in the corner. I knew what he was thinking: *Chick smokes some premium weed and flips out. Girl can't even hold her weed. What the fuck?*

Peter Frampton was playing. Jimmy sang, *Oooh, baby, I love your way—yesterday*. His friend laughed. Someone changed the record. The afternoon was slow, deadly. No one had anything to say. There was a party to get to and Jimmy had to go. No, he could not stay, impossible. His friend grunted goodbye. Wait up! Jimmy said. He kissed me on the cheek, turned back to his friend. See you, he said to me over his shoulder.

I feel the urge to write about the fear, anger, comic moments, and joy we experienced and hope this story may strike some familiar chords . . .

In pondering my mother's unfinished English paper, I wonder now about this notion of joy. I wonder it especially in relation to Jimmy. What was it that I felt? In retrospect, joy seems too easy, too unalloyed an emotion. Certainly I was happy to see him, ecstatic even. The sound of his voice on the phone could lift me from my gloom. I can remember laughing with him over silly things: leisure suits, TV commercials for air fresheners, the treacly messages of my Hallmark cards. Even now, all these years later, I recall details about him with a precision that borders on the uncanny. His untucked pink oxford shirt. His blue and white knit one. The one-handed way he removed his glasses before we settled in to kiss, the ironic way he tilted his head. Pink champagne, purple Cold Duck, red ceramic heart, yellow cheese; the colors of my world seemed heightened, perhaps because that world was so very small.

Jimmy, I knew, lived in the larger world and because of this I always knew we would part. Teen romances, of course, are fraught with the notion of parting; it's the common trope, the theme of countless radio ballads. Breaking up is hard to do. But what teenager ever begins a romance by envisioning its demise? We are, each of us, unique, that special case; we're going to be the ones to Make It, Find True Love, Beat the Odds. I knew better, and whatever joy I felt was tempered by this knowledge. At the time of my greatest isolation, Jimmy made me feel "normal." He made me, briefly, a coveted girl, someone cherished for herself. I know adults for whom this is difficult, who are uncomfortable around any kind of infirmity. The two or three times my father visited me at home he could not look me in the eye. *How long will you be sick?* How many times was I asked this? And here was Jimmy, wanting me to wash away perfume and artifice. I knew our relationship could never be sustained. We had drifted apart before we ever kissed, but these feelings were inchoate, difficult to express. Whatever joy I felt was suffused with the knowledge of our parting, a parting made no less painful by this awareness.

Meltings

Jimmy kept calling for a while after that last bad visit. We never spoke about the change in our relationship, but I knew we wouldn't be seeing each other anymore. Our conversations, so rambling and goofy, turned stilted. His grades were bad and his parents had begun talking about sending him to boarding school. If that happened he would run away to Florida. *Florida? Really?* I feigned disinterest. Since I could not say what I felt, I pretended to feel nothing. I met with my tutors, talked in the mornings to MJ or Sandy or Eileen, spent my afternoons with Betsy. The routine was incontrovertible.

Sunlight filled my room. The air turned sweet with flowers. My grandmother brought me lilac clippings that drooped from the weight of their own beauty, the branches trapped in crumpled foil. Their scent was overpowering. I had the shades kept pulled, the lilacs taken away. I could not stand their perfume, the spring breezes, the sounds of children playing. Winter, that great equalizer, had forced everyone indoors. Cocooned in my blankets, I'd merely been hibernating. Now I grew restless, something atavistic in the body needing to assert itself. I ached to move. The people around me began to wear summer clothes. Arms, calves, shoulders, all symmetrical and smooth. I hated the mildness and bounty of spring, which I felt as a rebuke to my condition.

The pain woke me from my nap. A new sensation, nothing to do with my spine. *My stomach*, I thought, though I'd eaten practically nothing. But . . . not my stomach, lower, a surging within my intestines. I felt nausea, cold sweats. *My appendix. They won't get to me in time; I'll die right here in this room.* Pain seeped from crevices, secret places. It was deep, deeper than bone. My muscles clenched, relaxed, tightened. I wanted to rub my stomach, curl into a ball, crawl under furniture, die. I wanted to die. I wanted to puke. I rang the bell, too late. Betsy cleaned me up, wiped my mouth, gave me sips of water. She sopped up the mess from the floor and spread an old rough towel over my pillow.

Show me where it hurts, she said. I pressed my palms to the cast. I didn't have words, didn't know. Down there? Not your stomach? I shook my head. She ripped some squares of toilet paper from the roll on my nightstand, showed me the chocolate smear of blood. Cramps, she said. I knew the term, had heard girls in homeroom: *I've got killer cramps!* Girls in the cafeteria explaining why they couldn't eat. They stood on two legs, brushed their hair, went to classes. Not like this.

A year earlier, when I was fourteen, I'd finally begun to menstruate. My mother had given me a box of Kotex, a new kind with adhesive strips—the greatest single invention of my youth. There would be no belt, no clanking of metal on fiberglass, no fumbling with clasps. In that regard at least I could assimilate, my body doing what it was supposed to do, not drawing attention to itself.

But after my surgery, my periods had stopped. Shock, I was told. This was normal, nothing to worry about. My system would adjust. Now, resurgent, my pent up period set me wailing. I rocked from side to side. The cramps came in waves. My mother had never mentioned cramps. For her they did not exist. In those days no one invoked PMS, the term was not yet in use. On TV commercials women spoke vaguely of the blues, but my mother had never experienced menstrual pain, mood swings, depression, thought these symptoms exaggerated, something in the head.

Betsy tore through the medicine cabinet. Midol, Pamprin . . . nothing. She gave me two aspirin and I puked them back up. I rolled and groaned; I wanted to double over, protect myself from the pain. Betsy changed the sheets. Because of the cast, none of my underwear fit. Even if it had, getting a pair on and off would have been a challenge for anyone and for this reason I went without. Somehow Betsy managed to jerry rig a pad to my mother's sanitary belt, which for some reason she had kept in the back of the linen closet, an emergency precaution. With some difficulty, Betsy was able to slide this contraption over my hips.

A week or so earlier, for Easter, Betsy had given me a basket with dyed eggs, chocolate eggs, jelly beans, a baggie of real grass tucked beneath pink artificial grass. Mild, she said, not to worry. We smoked a little and it eased the pain. When the blood came, all in a rush, I soaked through the pad and Betsy had to change it. I kept my face to the wall, ashamed. It was one more act of treason by a body I could never learn to trust.

Valium helped. Then it didn't. My prescription was switched to codeine. Then Seconal. Sleep was elusive. Barbiturate-stoned, I stopped dreaming, even that escape closed. There was only my room, the stereo, small television, silent telephone.

My mother came up with an idea. She would rent an ambulance, a private ambulance, to take me for a ride. Together we discussed the route. I had two hours, could go wherever I wanted. School was suggested. The ambulance could park in front and people could come out. I didn't want to go to school or any place public, didn't want to be on exhibit. Just drive around, I said. Drive around and I'll look out the window.

We chose an afternoon, a Saturday. We chose a route. My mother wrote it on a piece of paper that she gave to one of two uniformed attendants. They strapped me to a stretcher, brought me downstairs. The day was warm, the sun too bright. My eyes wet from it. Inside, the ambulance was cool and dark. An attendant covered me with blankets. My mother stayed with me; the attendants went up front. I could see out the window in the ambulance door. I watched the scenery—trees and steeples and telephone poles unspooling. We drove on back country roads and pulled over and an attendant opened the ambulance doors, letting the air rush in. Low stone fences, grassy hills, an abandoned well. Dogwoods and azaleas. The earth damp, reeking of peat. Birds swooped, branches swayed, clouds shifted, people walked, cars sped past, such exhausting motion. We drove to the beach and the salt air made me itch to be in the water. So long since I had felt water, the way it buoyed me, made me bodiless. We went to my friend Carol's house and her family came to the driveway and I wanted to see her brother Steve who had always been so attentive and gentle with me but he was not there. Later I discovered that she'd forgotten to tell him I was coming and he'd called her stupid and selfish and I was glad.

We drove and drove and I don't remember what the two hours felt like, whether fast or slow. When it was over and I was back in bed, I fell into a long sleep that did not need drugs to sustain it.

Don't you remember, though? There were two ambulance rides. The first one did you so much good that we scheduled a second one. We went back to the harbor and parked in a spot where you could see the water with the doors open. I don't think the second ride was as big a success. You already knew what to expect, and the long, drawn-out time of being in the cast, in bed, was really taking its toll.

I'm surprised when my mother insists that there were two ambulance rides. I have no recollection of this, or have somehow conflated the two trips.

The cast hurt so much you were crying. Probably you were suffering from "pressure sores," though I don't know if that's the correct technical term. Dr. Mangieri from the Bridgeport clinic made a house call, pretty unusual even in those days, but he was a nice guy and wanted, I think, to help when I told him how much pain you were having. He had a small drill and he put some holes in the cast to relieve the pressure, I think around your hip, maybe only one side.

You had this pointy chopstick you used to scratch yourself with. And you showed him, probably thinking he'd say how clever. But he frowned and told you to stop—not that you listened.

People were always coming in and out. Tom's nieces and nephews came to see you, and Carol and Janine, their boyfriends sometimes, and Betsy and her boyfriend, Frank; the university girls, Jimmy Hunter. I was always feeding someone. My mother gave me a microwave oven and I would defrost hotdogs. I know you won't eat them now, but back then you liked them.

After the cards and gifts stopped, after I grew used to my caretakers, after the snow melted and the weather turned warm, after Jimmy—especially after Jimmy—there is little specific that I recall. Of Dr. Mangieri's house call I have no memory whatsoever. I remember the hot dogs (now that my mother mentions them), and Betsy's boyfriend, Frank, stopping in to pick her up from work. But the steady flow of people in and out I suspect may be exaggerated. Many of them were likely single visits. It seems to me a great deal of my recuperation took place in solitude.

Some details, however, are remarkably clear. Faces close to mine, bodies leaning over me, kissing, tending, touching the exposed parts. A smell of lotion and powder, weed and piss. Betsy's little girl voice, MJ's bright blonde hair, the gold crucifix at her throat, Sandy's dark ponytail, her wine-colored birthmark, Mr. Dillon's aviator glasses, Mr. Martin's blushes, Jimmy's voice, still resonant. The pink walls of my bedroom, the pink phone and bedspread and mobile of abalone shells, all soon to disappear or be painted over white, to be obliterated, like memory. Entire swatches gone.

My father for instance. Where was he? I wrote that he visited me at home "two or three times," but this is because my mother says so. I have only a single recollection, when he could not look me in the eye, just as he'd been unable to in the hospital. My mother says there were two ambulance rides, not one; she says a doctor made a house call when the cast became too heavy; she says Dr. Syz, her taciturn Swiss boss, came over one Saturday to work on the Smithsonian catalogue for his Meissen porcelain collection. He came upstairs to say hello and when he returned, my mother says, He looked so incredibly sad, this man who was always so formal and reserved, never the least bit demonstrative. I could tell how moved he was, and it was all I could do to keep from crying.

I have no memory of his visit. I lay still, day after day, took barbiturates, watched TV. I read *Silas Marner* and *A Separate Peace* for Mr. Martin, memorized and forgot columns of irregular Spanish verbs. I counted weeks, months, then stopped counting. At best I would go directly from a plaster cast to a brace, bypassing the fiberglass body cast. At best I would be able to walk, and that was something huge. But my body would still be cloistered. There was to be no redemption—the princess set free, the duckling transformed into a swan, the frog to a prince, the authentic beautiful self bursting through the façade. Transformation was for fairy tales.

I woke one day, two or three weeks from the end, and could feel my body twitching. Like Mr. Dillon's rocks, my muscles strained to crack the crust under which they'd been trapped. In my carapace I shook and shook. My left leg thrashed and my arms flailed, hurling blankets to the floor, upsetting the water pitcher. My mother ran in to see what was wrong, but all I could say was Make It Stop. I couldn't do it any longer, lie still, not one day, not one hour. My body had been buried alive. Make it stop, I cried, just make it stop. She gave me a sedative. I came to, feeling calm. Everything was gray. Nighttime, but even with the light on the world seemed drained of color, as though I were viewing it through dark glasses. For some time—days? a week?—I did nothing at all. I refused to eat, wouldn't see my tutors, wouldn't do the work they assigned via my mother. I barely spoke. I lay in bed crying and saw the world as gray.

I had been the Statistic Gone Bad, the exception to every rule.

You'll exercise so you won't have to wear a brace, I'd been told.

You'll wear a brace so you won't undergo surgery.

You'll undergo surgery, but don't worry, eventually you'll be able to walk.

I wouldn't be able to walk. I was about to return to the hospital, and I was afraid.

Baby Steps

If everything went well I could leave the hospital within a week, sitting upright in my mother's Volkswagen.

It was difficult for me to believe that anything would go well. After the cast was removed I knew I would have to be x-rayed to make certain the fusion had stabilized. Although I no longer recall whether it was an actual or imagined possibility, I was terrified of being forced back into my cast and returned to my bed-tomb. There was as well the possibility, very slight, that I could skip the next step, the fiberglass "walking cast," and begin being weaned from the brace. I hated the brace. It was hot, hard, painful, and ugly. But it came off.

When I wasn't obsessing about being entombed in plaster, I permitted myself small moments in which I imagined my body set free. I pictured myself walking, running, tying my shoes. I wore a bathing suit, a midriff; I went swimming. Then I stopped. This was dangerous thinking. I told myself that the decision about what came next for me was not mine. I faked an attitude of calm. Que sera, sera; I knew that expression. Easy enough to sing on the A.M. radio, harder to adopt in a hospital. If everything was out of my hands (which it was) then there was nothing I could do (there wasn't), in which case it was pointless to worry (which I couldn't help doing). I merely needed to trust in my body, a thing I could not do.

One day after being admitted to the hospital, I was cut loose from my cast. Of the procedure itself, I remember only scattered details: the round saw slicing lines along my sides, spewing plaster dust; a gradual loosening of the plaster's grip along my torso, neck and thigh; a sense that I could breathe. The cast was removed in pieces, the top of the torso lifting like a giant lid, the bottom sliding from beneath me as I was maneuvered onto my side. I felt suddenly naked and cold. Layer after layer of dirty gauze and body stocking was peeled away. Goose bumps rose on my skin. I was a mummy being unwound. What would they find? The final layer of gauze was pulled off. My skin had turned it gummy and gray. For the first time in months I could see my stomach. It was ashen, mottled with pimples. My right thigh had purpled and shrunk to child size, smaller than my calves. I was turned onto my stomach. The scar was proclaimed beautifully healed. I had forgotten about the scar. I was desperate to scratch at my dirty flaky skin. A nurse washed me with an antibiotic soap, dried me with a rough towel. My skin thirsted for air. I was taken to be x-rayed, naked on the table. These x-rays would determine what would happen next. A mold was taken of my torso to fit a new brace. Then, just as I'd been after surgery, I was put into a kind of "holding cast," a plaster shell that covered my torso and prevented me from moving.

[Patient's] radiographs taken after removal of her cast demonstrated evidence of early bony fusion but motion was evident on bending films and thoracolumbar spine. The bony mass was likewise noted to be somewhat scant and it was decided to apply a light cast, body jacket with the neck left free and leg left free as well. A mold was taken for Milwaukee brace which she will wear after her light cast is removed.

—Dr. Wayne Southwick, Chief Orthopedic Surgeon
  Yale New Haven Hospital

Early mornings the hospital smelled of sausage, defrosted micro-waved breakfast sausage mingled with the sulfurous odor of boiled egg. I could never eat it, and this particular morning I could eat nothing at all. My mother and I waited for Dr. Southwick to make his rounds. She sat embroidering in the chair beside my bed while I looked at the ceiling-mounted television. Sometime in the late morning we heard Dr. Southwick's voice in the corridor. I turned off the TV. My mother put down her embroidery. She took hold of my hand. All of my resignation, my false sense of acceptance, evap-orated. I could not go back into the plaster cast. I'd beg, scream; I'd hoard barbiturates and overdose. I fully expected the news to be bad so when I saw the expression on Dr. Southwick's face—his broad smile, the way he extended his hand—I was more shocked than relieved. The news was not bad. The news, he said, was fine. My spine was fusing nicely. I was not yet ready to go back into my brace, but I could be switched into a fiberglass "walking" cast.

This new cast would extend from shoulder to hip; my neck and legs would be uncovered. Since fiberglass "breathed," I could take showers but not too often—two or three times a week. As soon as the cast was on, I could begin physical therapy and would be discharged once I could walk.

I heard the words "walk" and "cast" and they said to me two different, contradictory things. I was better, I could walk. I wasn't better, I'd have to remain in a cast for at least another three months. June, July, August . . . I'd be wrapped in fiberglass all summer. From the outset I had known that this was likely, but I'd done the forbidden thing—I'd allowed myself to imagine myself free. I was sick of casts, sick of being unable to see my body, rub my stomach when I had cramps, scratch my skin when it itched, sick of wear-ing ill-fitting clothes. I listened to Dr. Southwick, but my anguish prevented me from fully heeding his words. My mother rose to thank him. After he left, I vented: I wouldn't wear another cast, I was done with casts, tell them to come up with another plan, I was through! I'd roller-coasted from relieved—I could get out of bed—to resentful—this was never going to end! Each time I thought so, a new plan arose, exercise yielding to brace yielding to surgery. No, I said, I would not.

Despite my tirade, my mother was smiling, her eyes wet with tears.

You're going to walk, she said. Starting tomorrow.

I said I know and in saying that, I suddenly did know. Three months earlier I'd walked into the hospital. Since then I'd barely been able to move. My mother had devoted the past year almost exclusively to my care. She'd gone to work, come home, gone directly to my room to see what I needed. She'd dealt with doctors, nurses, interns, technicians, trying her best to shield me from those who were impatient and brusque. Weekends, evenings, she'd spent in the hospital, sometimes sleeping beside me in a chair. She'd prayed and cursed, probably in the same stream of breath. She'd fired one nurse and had found for me a friend in another; she'd convinced a doctor to come to our home and ambulance attendants to take me on joy rides. Most likely she'd neglected her husband and son, something I'd never considered. And now it was about to end. I was, I finally realized, not the only one who was going to be liberated.

I know, I said. Meaning I would walk, meaning so much more than that, not having the words for it, hoping that she knew.

The new cast looked like the top half of a pair of overalls, but with wide shoulder straps. My torso was again wrapped in a body stocking to which thick layers of fiberglass were applied. Once again a shell separated me from my body. I watched myself being covered up, the mummy returning to the crypt. Silently I said goodbye to my torso. Goodbye, see you in three months.

This cast was lighter than the plaster one, lighter even than the brace. For the first time in nearly three years my head and neck were free. I could not yet move them, nor sit up, but I stared at my neck in the hand mirror, imagining how it would look adorned with necklaces, silk scarves, Jimmy's red ceramic heart. A long thin neck, like a ballerina's I'd been told, and I pictured myself in a white tutu, curtseying onstage, as I was presented with dozens of long-stemmed roses.

I was strapped to a table, the kind you see in Frankenstein movies when the monster is about to be set upright and loosed upon the world. A physical therapist began by degrees to tilt the table, stopping every so often so I could get used to each new position. Breathe deeply, she counseled, as though we were in the High Himalayas. Twenty degrees, thirty. My head grew light. Miles below I could see my feet in their spongy blue hospital slippers. Forty-five degrees. The blood rushed from my head. My feet disappeared. I feel faint, I said, and when I came to I was supine.

The next day I held at forty-five degrees, though I again felt lightheaded. I gripped the table and vowed not to faint. Slowly the therapist tilted the table. Slowly I made my vertical ascent. I shut my eyes, took deep breaths. I was spinning through space. Purple circles swirled behind my eyes. The table went completely upright. I was vertical. I blacked out. The therapist lowered the table, but not all the way. She did this, raising and lowering the table for most of the afternoon, until I could stay upright.

Because I was too weak to walk I was moved from my bed to a wheelchair. In the evenings, after therapy, I'd tool up and down the main corridor of the adolescent ward, giddy with mobility. Sometimes I'd wheel into the patients' lounge, where a cherubic looking boy in a leg cast held long make-out sessions with his girlfriend. The boy had been hurt in a motorcycle accident and confined to bed. His girlfriend wore tight jeans, big hoop earrings, her long hair streaked blonde. Whenever she wanted to be alone with her boyfriend, which was pretty much always, she'd snap her fingers and say, We're busy in here! Cowed, the other patients would leave. When she wasn't there the boy would talk to us about his accident, showing off the burns on his other leg. Nothing wrong with me, he'd say. I ain't sick, not like some people here.

The other patients and I would watch TV, which we could do as well in our rooms. But in this common space we were able to check each other out, see who was in for what and how long, who had it better—or worse—than we did.

I missed Jimmy. Every day I thought about calling him. He didn't know I was in the hospital. Maybe he'd come see me. But I knew that even were he to say yes, which was unlikely, things between us would be strained. He had brought his friend as a buffer. He'd sung those lyrics about me. I wanted the initials he'd carved—my initials—to scar his arm. We would be marked by this time—the pencil line down my back, the fading welts of my initials linking us.

My roommate this time around was in for a nose job. She had a deviated septum, wore a plaster over her nose, and for some reason had to take her meals through a straw. A year older than me, she had a boyfriend and at night she'd talk to him on the phone, giggling the hours away. Her parents felt sorry for me, I could tell. They brought us both milkshakes and they looked at me with that expression of pity I'd grown used to. They saw the wheelchair, the body cast; of course they did, who wouldn't? They saw me, the disabled girl. But they did not see what I had been. I could go where I wished now and soon I would begin to walk. Disability was a way station and I was a person in transit. People saw me differently from others, I knew that. But I was beginning to see myself differently, too.

Before I could walk I had to learn to stand. Before I could stand I had to build up my muscles. I spent hours in therapy, stretching my legs, lifting them, bending, strengthening my atrophied thigh. I moved my head from side to side. The brace had held my neck in place for over two years before it was cemented into the cast, and my range of motion was small. From lack of use my arms were weak. Every muscle had gone slack. The therapist and I worked all afternoon. By bedtime I was always exhausted, sleeping through the night without chemical intervention.

My lessons in walking began at the parallel bars. The therapist helped hoist me from my wheelchair. I kept my weight in my left leg, which was stronger from not having been in a cast, and held onto to the bars, my arms shaking. I'd been off my feet for so long that I needed to keep my head down until my vision cleared. For a while I stood at the entrance to the parallel bars, getting used to the familiar new sensation of standing, my weight in my left leg, my right foot skimming the floor. My shoulders rolled forward and my neck felt floppy, too insubstantial to support my head. I didn't think my legs would hold up and I was afraid of falling, of damaging the spinal fusion, breaking something, being returned to bed.

At the therapist's direction I shifted my weight bit by bit into my right leg, still clutching the bars. Pins and needles pricked my foot. I shifted back, taking all of my weight into my good leg. The therapist urged me on. *Again! Keep trying.* This time the pain was worse, needles shooting up my leg, like whacking my funny bone on the edge of the kitchen table. *Let go now. Let go of the bars.* The prospect of letting go terrified me. I held fast to the bars. The therapist was standing beside me and she promised to catch me if I began to fall. We had to start sometime, she said. Didn't I want to go home? I was scared, but I did as she said; I let go. My right knee buckled and I grabbed bars. *Good! Again!* Good? I'd nearly fallen. Both my legs ached and we'd just begun. I wanted to sit down. I couldn't even stand; how was I ever to walk? All afternoon the therapist coached me: shift weight, let go, stand. When my right knee gave way, I clung to the bars until, by the end of the session, I could keep weight in that leg without holding on. I favored my left leg and still do, so that even in recent photos I can be seen leaning markedly to the left. But I could keep both feet on the floor, unsupported.

The next day we practiced baby steps. I set my right foot down lightly, with great precision. To walk I would need to put all of my weight into that leg, which was not yet strong enough to support me, so I held onto the bars. The therapist stood beside me, cajoling. *Let go. Take a step.* I did, wobbling, steadying myself. I was a toddler, a big unsteady toddler, learning to walk. *Great! Another!* We went on like this. I could take only a step or two before I had to grab the bars, "walking" with my arms, which began to ache from the strain. I had never been an athlete, never been able to bike or hike or run very far, but at least I had been able to take walking for granted, and now I was frustrated, my steps so tiny and painful and slow. My grandfather, with his Parkinson's disease, walked better than this. But his disability could arc in only one direction, toward immobility, while mine I knew was slowly moving in the other direction. Eventually I would walk.

I traded up, from wheelchair to walker. Instead of cruising along the adolescent ward's main corridor I shuffled, just as I'd seen those elderly patients do in physical therapy all those years ago, leaning into their walkers, chatting about their grandchildren while I exercised my back muscles so that I wouldn't have to wear a brace.

I could stand. I could get in and out of bed. I could use the bathroom by myself. But I could not walk unassisted, and I could not yet go home.

The motorcycle boy and his girlfriend were making out in the lounge. My roommate and I stayed in our room watching TV together. Earlier in the day I'd had therapy and I was tired and sore. I needed to use the bathroom, always a chore because with the walker I was so slow. The wheelchair had been so much faster. Little by little, I eased myself from my chair, holding tightly to the walker. I'd managed so far to walk the length of the parallel bars but had been unable to let go. I wanted to walk, to go home. I shuffled toward the bathroom then stopped and turned my walker to the wall. When I reached the wall I slumped against it, leaning on my right shoulder. All my weight was in my left leg. I pressed my palms and shoulder to the wall, shifted my weight and took a step. As soon as my left foot touched the floor I lifted my other foot and let go of the wall. Another step. Leaned back into the wall as my right foot came down, using my fingertips for support. Another step. Leaned back into the wall. My roommate stood nearby, ready to catch me if necessary, but she did not interfere. Another baby step. With great deliberation I made my way to the bathroom. Another step, right foot. Left foot, my fingertips tracing the wall. Right foot. Left foot, no hands, just my shoulder against the wall. Right foot. Left foot and this time I did not touch the wall. I was walking, unencumbered.

Partings

I wanted to touch everything, see, smell, feel everything. I'd sit in the yard wearing only a pair of denim cut-offs because the cast covered my torso. Arms, legs, feet, neck bare to the sun, I scooped dirt by the handful, sifted it through my fingers, twisted clovers into rings, braided blades of grass with my spittle. I was too weak to leave home, too unsteady to stay long on my feet. Through the end of May the university girls came in the mornings to care for me. Each week I grew a little stronger and by the end of the month I could go on short trips. MJ drove us to her family's beach cottage, a shabby-chic place in a row of identical cottages where university students crashed, six or eight to a cottage, and threw raucous keg parties that I aspired to attend. She helped me up the porch steps and through the back door. The curtains were drawn, the cottage dark. It smelled of Pine Sol and the sea, a smell I loved. Her grandmother said hello and help yourself. She seemed not the least bit curious about me or surprised by my appearance so I assumed they must have discussed me before. MJ made tuna sandwiches and iced tea. She helped me onto the sand where she spread a blanket so we could eat. She'd changed into a bikini; I wore my cut-offs and an oversized T-shirt. I was allowed to wade up to my knees but knew I could not withstand even the gentlest current and so stayed on the blanket looking at the water, smelling the salt air, feeding crusts to the gulls, watching them swoop and scatter.

A pan of water had been placed by the back door for rinsing sand off one's feet. I stepped into it, an ablution. The water was grainy and warm. I looked down at my legs, scrawny, Renaissance white, like those paintings of Jesus I'd seen in art class. I went to the bathroom mirror. My cheeks were hollow, my eyes unusually large, a spray of freckles across my nose from the recent sun. I had no idea what I weighed because I had no idea what the cast weighed. But I was skinny, even with the added weight. I could feel my hip bones, unpadded, jutting against the cast, could feel the pressure on my stomach. I'd eaten half the tuna sandwich; I ate all my meals by halves. The era of the Big Model had begun, the big-haired athletic girl, Farrah and Jaclyn with their muscles and teeth. And I could not stand at the water's edge for fear of being toppled. There was no way to be other than what I was.

Afternoons Betsy came and we watched TV downstairs on the big set and sometimes she took me on errands—to the dry cleaners or bank or grocery store. I was happy to go anywhere. Sometimes we went back to her apartment and sometimes other people were there—Frank, his friends, and we sat around and played records and smoked, and sometimes Frank cooked spaghetti and I'd call my mother and say I was staying for dinner. I felt grown up among these people in their twenties, people with apartments and jobs, though I knew I was only a spectator of their lives.

Eileen and Sandy were returning to New Jersey. MJ was taking a vacation. My mother decided I no longer needed help in the mornings, especially given how late I slept. She bought wine and crackers, paté, cheeses and threw a farewell party. She put money in cards for the girls who, in turn, had brought me gifts of jewelry. Eileen had graduated and would not be back, but MJ and Sandy each had another year to go. We'll see you in the fall, they said. We'll stop by, we'll visit. We hugged goodbye, all of us crying, believing the words, yet knowing how unlikely they were.

I did not want Betsy to go. She couldn't stay, she had to work, my mother could not pay her to watch TV and be my friend. But

I'm still weak, I protested. You see how long it takes me to get up these stairs? What if there's an emergency?

Call 911, she said.

She agreed to have Betsy come two afternoons a week until she found a new job. I didn't want this to happen. It won't be like here, I warned. They'll make you wear a uniform. They won't let you smoke pot. Betsy took hold of my hand. She knew, she said, but what was to be done? We had to get on with our lives. I could walk. Every day I was stronger. By fall I wouldn't even need the cast. Wasn't that what I wanted? I nodded, but felt confused. What I wanted was for her—not just her, but especially her—to stay in my life, even as I was beginning to realize how impossible that was.

We'll stay friends, Betsy promised, and for a while this was true. She'd pick me up after work, still in her uniform, and bring me home for dinner. She took me to a Yes concert and we sat on a hill sharing a bottle of Riunite and watching the laser show. But she was ten years older than me and had the life of an adult, an insuperable barrier.

School ended, the university girls went away. Betsy got a new job. The weather turned hot. Beneath the cast I could feel my skin shed. I clawed at fiberglass, a corset of emery board. The brace had been more restrictive than the cast, heavier, but because I could remove it, I'd been able to wash. Now I felt sticky all the time.

Three days a week, during the hottest part of the afternoon, I stood beneath the shower's spray, letting cool water stream inside the cast. I dried in the sun until the heat became too much then aimed the hair dryer nozzle down into the cast with the setting on low so my skin wouldn't burn. I imagined gauze soaking up water, sweat, turning to moss. I dumped Johnson's Baby Powder through the armholes of the cast, spilling talcum on the bathroom floor, where it gummed to a paste.

Because the cast could not be removed, I needed underwear that would fit over it, giant cotton underwear—pink, blue, white— the kind my grandmother wore, another indignity.

Day after day I lay on the couch, a slug. At night my mother would take Chipper and me to Baskin-Robbins or Dairy Queen, coax me to eat. I'd finish half a chocolate-dipped cone, give the rest to Chipper, who'd already devoured a banana split. Night became the only time I would go outside. We'd stand beneath the Dairy Queen's humid yellow glow, cones dripping, insects buzzing, my mother saying *One more bite.* I was a disabled vampire, feeding on ice cream instead of blood.

Jimmy called. He wanted to see me, could he come visit? I was wanting, wary—wanting to think my walking would make a difference, wary about his motives. He must have known I was out of bed. Did he think me "cured?"

I'm still in a cast, I warned. It's smaller than the other one and I can walk but it's still a body cast.

I was giving him a chance to change his mind. He didn't take it. Because he was still in school he'd come on Saturday. That too made me anxious. If he came on a weekday we could be alone. But skipping school meant a short visit, not an overnight. He said he'd hitch down, not trouble my mother—a way of remaining noncommittal.

Saturday I waited in the living room so I could be first at the door, greet him, and go straight upstairs, not stopping to chat with my mother or Tom. Jimmy had said afternoon, and I began my vigil just after twelve. I sat on the couch, facing the window. The chair, a wing back upholstered in a faded pattern of blue and gold flowers, would have been more comfortable. It had a matching ottoman and offered better back support. But Tom had claimed the chair for himself and no one, not even my mother, was allowed to sit in it. Perhaps for that reason it was my favorite place to read, and I sat there many weekday afternoons while Tom was at work.

Two, three hours, I waited. I tried to read. Every half hour I checked the kitchen clock. Finally, mid-afternoon, Jimmy arrived. I took him to my room, leaning heavily on the banister, propelling myself upstairs as fast as I could. Jimmy took the desk chair; I sat stiffly on the edge of my bed, a single bed, pushed into a corner. The hospital bed and table had been returned to the supply store, and all the paraphernalia of my recovery—bedpan, bed tray, pitcher, shampoo board, bell—had been removed. My room looked bigger now, just another bedroom, and I'd decided to paint it white. I told Jimmy that, struggling for things to say. He came and sat beside me. I was taller by at least two inches, forced by my fusion to sit upright. I leaned toward him, stiffly, needing to bend. It was difficult for him to get his arms around the cast. We kissed. He kept his glasses on, a screen. Downstairs we could hear a commotion, Tom yelling at my mother for me to open the door. I wanted it like before, with the cold and dark at the window and us buried in blankets, three in the morning, drifting off to sleep. But it was sunny and hot, my body itched inside the fiberglass, and Tom was downstairs yelling *Open the God damned door!*

Jimmy said, No way your mother's gonna let me sleep in here tonight. The thought that we would be separated, that he would be exiled to another room, had never occurred to me. This was Jimmy. We'd slept together before. I was in a cast, a full body cast, my breasts, stomach, and hips covered in fiberglass.

No, I insisted, she'll let you, I know. He gave me that skeptical look, eyebrows raised, I'd seen whenever we'd made fun of something, only nothing was funny this time. I wanted to kiss him again, but he pulled away.

You'll see, he warned.

To escape the yelling we went outside. I was too weak to leave the yard. I wished that one of us was older, had a car, could get away, to Florida like he'd wanted, the Green Comet Diner, anywhere.

My mother called us in for dinner. Jimmy sat next to me, with Tom at one end of the table and my mother at the other. Across from me Chipper wolfed his food, one hand on his milk glass, the other shoveling. Slow down, Tom said. No one's going to take it away. He grilled Jimmy about his father, the judge. I knew this impressed him, his own father having been a judge, and I thought him stupid and snobbish but I doubt there was anything he could have said or done that I would not have resented. Who was he to me, this man incapable of a kind word or gesture? He paid the bills, that was all. *You're not my father!* I'd yell, unable to acknowledge that this was precisely the point, the reason my mother had married him. My father was living in a Manhattan high-rise with an East River view, a parking garage, girlfriends. He neglected to pay child support; he forgot our birthdays. I knew this, yet every day I wished Tom gone from our lives and only felt at ease when he was away.

Jimmy answered Tom's questions. I tried to make eye contact—*Isn't this stupid, I know they're stupid*—but he wouldn't take the bait. After dinner we returned to my room. Keep the door open, my mother said. Not all the way, but not closed either. Halfway. This was her compromise. I was shocked. In front of Jimmy she had taken Tom's side, betraying me and proving Jimmy right.

With the door open we had to keep the music down and could not smoke pot. I was self-conscious about our conversation, not knowing what to say, not wanting to be overheard. I knew Tom capable of eavesdropping; he'd complained to my mother when I'd stayed up all night on the phone with Jimmy. *They don't even talk about anything, they just ramble.* For about the millionth time, I wished him dead.

We went back outside and that was not much better since we could be seen from both the kitchen and from my mother's bedroom. The shade was down, though, and we risked sharing a pipe. We sat on a picnic bench in the dark, not talking, and it wasn't like our earlier silences when we'd been happy and sated. We both knew this visit was a mistake, one we were stuck with until morning.

At 11:00 I was told to go to bed. I'd never had a bedtime, my arrangement with my mother being that if I stayed on the Honor Roll I could go to bed when I liked. Jimmy was banished to the couch in the den, another betrayal. Always before, my mother had taken my side against Tom; it was something I could count on. Now, suddenly, she was acting as if she could not trust me and because of that, because she had ruled in favor of her husband, I no longer felt I could entirely trust her. Despite my body cast, Jimmy and I were not to be left alone. The implications were insulting; I felt them less, I think, on my own behalf than on his. A boy who had always changed his clothes in the bathroom. Who had done nothing more physical than kiss me, said nothing more insinuating than "honey." Once during the night I tried to sneak downstairs. My mother heard me, said, Don't try it again, not if you don't want to be grounded. As a concept, "grounded" was meaningless—where would I have gone? But I didn't want a scene. I stayed in my room fiddling with the antenna of the black and white TV that had been returned to me in exchange for the color set, trying to tune in *Saturday Night Live.* The picture stayed fuzzy and after a while I gave up.

Jimmy left in the morning. I knew that he would not come back. I saw him once more, about a year later, in the fall of my senior year. He'd spent the previous year in boarding school. We'd never said goodbye, never exchanged letters; I hadn't even known he was gone. When he called me I was so surprised that he had to say his name twice.

Skip school, he said. Skip school tomorrow and come to New York and we'll go to museums. Museums? This too was a surprise. We'd never discussed art. I was unsophisticated, knew little about paintings, had never been in New York without some supervising adult.

He could have said "baseball," which bored me to a near narcoleptic state. Or opera or rodeo. Could have said we'll ride the subway all day or sit in the station watching the trains go by. None of it would have mattered.

Since I'd last seen him my cast had come off. I'd stopped wearing the brace, even at night. Strangers who saw me had no idea. Jimmy had no idea. I didn't tell him. It would be a surprise—See, this is me, my real self. A spell would be lifted; we'd have a happy ending after all.

I was of course too smart or dubious or pessimistic to really believe this, but I wanted his approval, his look of shocked delight. At last we would be evenly matched, two inconspicuous kids playing hooky, nothing remarkable about them at all.

I told my mother I had First Period study hall. It may have been true. Seniors were not required to attend study hall and my mother agreed to let me drive her to work then take her VW to school so I wouldn't have to walk home. I was to pick her up at 5:00, which meant I needed to be back at the train station by 4:30. The trip to New York took seventy minutes. Jimmy rode in from New Haven and I met him, as arranged, in the last car. I knew he would be on the train, but he stepped briefly onto the platform to let me know he'd made it.

Jimmy looked the same. He said nothing about my appearance; his face showed no surprise. I'd expected . . . what? Astonishment, accolades—*My God, look at you, so beautiful, who knew, what a dope I've been!* A word or two of recognition, some look. But it was as though nothing had changed, which meant that everything had.

We made small talk. We knew no one in common, his new school was in another state, there was none of the easy mindless banter that connects people of long acquaintance. For seventy minutes we struggled to fill the trip with words.

Grand Central Station in 1977 was a neglected, shabby place. Turquoise paint flaked from the ceiling of the Great Hall; people slept on benches in the Vanderbilt Lobby, begged for change outside the scarred wooden doors of the ladies' room stalls. Some of the windows were still blacked out from World War II. A vast illuminated Kodak ad beamed down from the mezzanine: wide-toothed blonde children cavorting in the orange foliage. Still I was struck, as always, by the majesty of the station, its vastness, its balconies and double staircases, the constellations splayed on the vaulted ceiling. I lingered, staring at the mustard-hued stars: horse and hunter and crab.

But Jimmy was in a hurry. There were museums to get to, time was short; he hustled us into the taxi queue and we rode up to the Met, each of us looking out our separate window.

Jimmy paid the fare. He knew exactly where to go, which rooms, which paintings, knew how much admission to pay, not the "suggested price" but not nothing, something in-between.

I had been with my family to the lobby of the Met to see the Christmas tree, along with the grander tree at Rockefeller Center and the Rockettes at Radio City Music Hall. I'd never been inside the museum proper, though. Jimmy led the way down long corridors with scuffed parquet floors to a room of bright paintings. Ballerinas, lily pads, haystacks, flowering trees and gardens in elaborate gold frames. *Impressionism.* I did not know the word. *Look.* Jimmy took my hand and brought me inches from a painting composed entirely of dots. *Pointillism. Now stand back. See?* The dots massed into solid shapes: a woman, a parasol, a monkey, tiny background sailboats. I scanned the identifying plaque, hoping for clues. *Ser-aht.* I said the painter's name aloud. A "study" by "Ser-aht." Gently Jimmy corrected me. *Ser-ah, not Ser-aht. Georges Seurat.* I mimicked the way he said it. I didn't know what else to say. I told him I thought Pointillism was "cool."

We spoke softly, the rooms quiet, nearly empty. In another room flat beige paintings, figures assembled from squares. Picasso, whose name I recognized, and someone named Braque. *Cubism.* I'd heard the term, but the paintings confused me. How had they been made—and why? *Why are they like this?* I could tell he thought it a stupid question.

Up Fifth Avenue, along Central Park, we walked to the Guggenheim. A weekday in October, the park was hushed, sunlight filtered through the arcade of trees. People strolled, we strolled. I thought how lovely to live here and walk in this park and go to these museums whenever one wished, and I told Jimmy I wanted to live here some day and asked did he and he said no, it's way too crowded.

In the Guggenheim more paintings of cubes and dots, and other paintings that were a single color—red or black or white.

I didn't understand these at all, didn't know what to think. Minimalism, he called it, and I was afraid to ask. Gradually we spiraled up the ramp, making detours into side rooms, so that I was surprised to see how far we'd gone when we reached the top. Far below us was the lobby floor, polished and white, the base of Mount Everest. *Look*, I wanted to shout, *Look what I just did!* but it was only an everyday occurrence.

For lunch we ate hamburgers at a diner, splitting the tab. Nearly two years earlier I'd fantasized about dimly lit restaurants, candles and wine, images culled from old movies. Jimmy devoured his burger, I picked at my fries. The lights were harsh, the silverware spotted, we had to rush to catch our train.

When we got to the Fairfield station, just ahead of the evening commuters, he gave me a perfunctory kiss, stepping from the car for a moment before the train doors shut.

What had he wanted, what had prompted him to call? Idle curiosity? Did he want to see what I had become? Or was it more complicated than that? Beneath the teenage swagger was a reticence. This was someone after all who'd chosen, albeit briefly, to be with a girl whose body he could not see. A girl for whom physical intimacy had been impossible. Something had held him back. Now that I was "normal," he didn't try to touch me, nor did he comment on the change. Other boys did, asking me out, pressuring me to sleep with them. The boy in Social Studies who stared at my legs and told me I should wear short skirts. The boy who, while dating a friend of mine, had barely spoken to me but now wanted to know if I would come over when his father was away. The ones who asked to copy my homework, saying *Patti, you're so smart*, as though they had just noticed and were turned on by my brains. The men in parking lots who whistled. I didn't want any of them. Their urgency frightened me, their desire to touch. For so long I'd been invisible. Now I wanted to be noticed, but became flustered when I was. I felt unequipped to flirt, didn't know the language, the rules involved, watched the other girls twirl their hair, swap notes, raise and lower their eyelids, one more exam I was studying for, harder than my other exams.

Jimmy didn't see me through a sexual lens, which puzzled me because it seemed as if suddenly everyone else did. Even my mother had not let me be alone with him once I could walk. It was as though in shedding the apparatus of brace and cast I'd shed the person I had been. I had thought I wanted this, wanted to be seen for myself, but now I realized I didn't know what that meant. Hadn't I been "myself" all along? If people hadn't noticed me, if what they'd seen was instead the brace, could I honestly say they were seeing me now? I'd been metal, plaster, and fiberglass; now I was breasts and hips, just another girl, just what I had wanted and could not bear. I hadn't traded one self for another, a nun for a vamp, and this abrupt shift in the perspective of others was something that I struggled to understand.

Pacifying the Beast

X-rays show an excellent position. Patient should change over to her brace now and go out of it one hour a week until about October, at which time she can wear it only to sleep in all probability. She is to come back in October for new x-rays.

—Dr. Wayne Southwick, Chief Orthopedic Surgeon
Yale New Haven Hospital

Breasts, hips, stomach, ribs. I could not stop staring. My body had been given back to me. In the afternoons, when my mother and Tom were at work, I'd take off my clothes and look at myself in the full-length mirror on their bedroom door. My bones were nearly visible beneath the netting of skin, my waist small from confinement. I counted ribs, traced hipbones, clavicles, Twiggy at last.

The members of my family were big-boned, robust people who seemed to take their bodies for granted. Rather then seeing myself as thin, I saw their bulkiness, the encumbrance of flesh. That was my bias, viewed through a distorted lens, just as it had been difficult for the able-bodied to clearly see me. I was "poor thing." I was Robot and Monkey and Turtle; eventually I became Baby, another generic girl whose substitute name was shouted from passing cars.

By fall I was only wearing the brace to sleep. During the day nothing marked me as different; no one knew. Weeknights my mother strapped me in before midnight; weekends I had to be home by that hour so she could corset me. This curfew applied to her as well; she had to leave parties early to help me into the brace. Don't worry, I'd say. No big deal, just tonight, stay out late, have fun. A waste of breath. If my mother resented this imposition on her freedom she didn't let it show. A small matter after all we'd been through, but I was impatient, sick of waking during the night with the weight of metal on my back, angry at this transformation into a visibly disabled person—even if no one could see.

For Christmas the previous year I'd been given a copy of Thomas Bulfinch's *Mythology*. The book was heavy, bound in deep blue faux-leather, thickly illustrated, too heavy for me to hold above my head all those months I was supine. By summer—Jimmy gone, the university girls returned home, Betsy working another job—I was spending most of my time alone. The fiberglass cast was hot in the sun. I turned my air-conditioner to ten, wrapped myself in blankets, and read Bulfinch, revisiting the Greek myths I loved, skimming through the Norse section (all that ice, those horned helmets and animal skins), lingering at the Arthurian tales. In particular I liked the story of Dame Ragnell, who tricks King Arthur into getting her way.

According to Bulfinch, Dame Ragnell was "a lady of hideous aspect" whom King Arthur happens upon in the forest. The lady confronts him, asking by what right he refuses to look at her when she, in fact, possesses what he has been seeking—the answer to the question: "What thing is it that women most desire?" If the king cannot answer this riddle within a year, he must forfeit his life and lands to the evil baron who has posed the question. The year is nearly up. Dame Ragnell promises to answer the riddle—in exchange for marriage to Sir Gawain, the king's nephew.

King Arthur is reluctant to condemn his nephew to such a fate, marriage to a hag. Her skin is coarse, her hair bristling, her teeth yellow and sharp. What would she be like to touch? But Gawain insists on saving his sovereign's life. They accept Dame Ragnell's terms. "Women," she tells the king, "would have their will."

King Arthur repeats this answer to the evil baron, the curse is lifted, and Sir Gawain marries the "loathly lady" in a ceremony devoid of festivities while his companions "scoffed and jeered." Yet that night, alone with her husband in the bridal chamber, Dame Ragnell, to Gawain's amazement and delight, sheds her "unseemly aspect" to reveal her true form: a beautiful young maiden. She explains to the astonished Gawain that she'd been under a spell, condemned to appear hideous until two things occurred. The first was that some gallant knight consent to marry her. This being accomplished, half the curse has been lifted and she is free to wear her true form for half of the time. Gawain is to choose: should she be fair by day or night?

Sir Gawain would fain have had her look her best by night, when he alone would see her, and show her repulsive visage, if at all, to others. But she reminded him how much more pleasant it would be to her to wear her best looks in the throng of knights and ladies by day. Sir Gawain yielded, and gave up his will to hers. This alone was wanting to dissolve the charm. The lovely lady now with joy assured him that she should change no more, but as she now was, so she would remain by night as well as by day.

Having broken the spell, Dame Ragnell, beloved of Gawain, is accepted at court. The jeers and taunting cease. Gawain is a happy man, Ragnell a happy woman.

Now that I, too, was free to reveal my "true form" during the day, I couldn't stop wondering at the change in those around me. The jeers and taunting stopped. Popular girls deigned to speak to me. Boys asked about parties, weekend plans. My mother became more watchful, my brother less solicitous. We fought, yelled, insulted each other like ordinary siblings. He hung out in my room again listening to music and threatening to tell my mother that I smoked pot, a threat we both recognized as empty.

Disabled people freak people out, he'd said, explaining why my condition had made him uneasy. But it goes deeper than that. Visible difference freaks people out. Nonconformity, in any guise, is a potential threat.

In the early 1990s, in Boston, a spate of gay bashing occurred near my place of work. My boss, a deeply religious black woman, expressed her dismay, claiming it was wrong to "pick on" gay people. *They just can't help the way they are. It's like picking on the crippled.* When I suggested that gay people might not consider themselves "crippled," that they may, in fact, have no more wish to be straight than she did to be white, she recoiled. Surely no one would choose to flout, so visibly, the mores of the crowd. Homosexuality was a "disease," like polio, something to be pitied, something that allowed her to make a show of her tolerance. I'd spent my adolescence deflecting this adult tolerance—strangers who clucked their tongues, called me "dear," and felt free to interrogate me. Pointing children, apologetic mothers, their smiles watery and sad. People who spoke of faith healers or invoked the will of God, infuriating my mother, who'd heard the same phrase years ago, when her first child had died.

My boss pitied the people under attack but she could not make the difficult leap from tolerance to acceptance. For Dame Ragnell acceptance came with the lifting of a spell, for me with the removal of a brace. But self-acceptance proved a more complicated matter than I'd imagined.

From my high school journal:
Got home in an awful mood. Out of money, the house a mess and to top it all off, my stomach screaming "Feed me! Feed me, you sadistic fool. It's 2:30, and you haven't fed me since dinner last night." Terrible pest, the stomach. I stuck a bar of frozen cream cheese in the microwave to pacify the beast. Three minutes later I had a plate full of mushy molten mess. My eyes took one look at it, and my stomach instantly stopped its incessant screaming. That'll teach it!

Breakfast was coffee with sugar and milk. Lunch a Dannon yogurt or a three-pack of chocolate chip cookies. I hoarded my lunch money, went in on ounce bags with my new friends, kids who took classes in writing and art. We huddled outside, cupped our hands around the joint, kept watch for the assistant headmaster, who wore pastel leisure suits and could be spotted in time for one last hit before someone stomped out the roach and I popped a breath mint, dessert.

Dinner was compulsory. I wanted to eat, but my appetite remained static. Still I was expected to eat the same amount as everyone else, my "May I Please Be Excused?" answered with "Not Until You Finish What's On Your Plate." My mother's rejoinders were anxious, Tom's punitive, but they amounted to the same thing. I cut tiny pieces, swallowed them whole and cold, soldiering my way through collapsed vegetables, unctuous potatoes, meat that leaked blood. I wanted salads, juices, air. I was afraid of growing big, like those field hockey girls with their bulging calves and mannish shoulders. At night, bracing me, my mother would tug on the leather strap, pulling it as far as it would go, buckling the corset at the tightest hole. The brace shifted, loose on my hips. My body was the enemy; made strong, there was no telling what havoc it might cause. I didn't think this, not rationally, but my mistrust of my physical needs ran deep, as my journal attests. So I shaped myself into a blade.

Had I known the repercussions of this behavior, I might have made an effort to feed myself. Instead I starved my bones of all they needed—exercise, sunlight, nutrients. Partly this was unavoidable. One can't exercise when one cannot move; nor, encased in metal or fiberglass, can one linger in the sun, nor eat much when corseted in plaster. Muscles and appetite shrink, lethargy takes hold. Still I suppose that, once unbound, I'd have tried to replenish my bones instead of starving my body to "get even" with it.

But perhaps not. I was self-absorbed, immersed in the present, which is to say I was a teenager. The future was too distant to hold sway. Even if I'd been able to fathom it, to gauge the consequences of my actions, I might not have changed a thing. My distrust of my body was a force resistant to reason.

A new year, and I was healed at last. People who hadn't known me before, what did they know? During exams doctors admired my scar—so thin, so light. Its beauty lay in its near invisibility. To heal meant to fade. I would fade like my scar, be made thin like my scar, the ultimate synecdoche.

I needed new clothes, ones tailored to my body not my brace. My mother took me shopping, making an event of it, going from store to store—elegant little Westport boutiques, a Fairfield strip mall, a hippie emporium behind a beaded curtain in an ice cream parlor with marble-topped tables and nickelodeons that showed *The Bum's Rush* and *The Perils of Pauline*. We splurged on ice cream in silver dishes, a single scoop I struggled to finish. Fed our change to the nickelodeons, turning the crank to see the train bearing down on Pauline as the hero galloped to her rescue. I knew she'd be saved, yet I savored the menace. So different, these excursions, from the ones we'd made a year earlier, sitting gloomy and silent in the Rathskeller after another hospital visit.

My new clothes were showy, but showed little of me. After years of being hidden, I felt suddenly exposed. My hated brace had nonetheless protected me from the predatory gaze. It had desex-ualized me, made me "safe," the chaperone on other girls' dates, the sidekick. Because of this I was unprepared in many ways for its removal. Freedom, comfort, I yearned for these things. But it was more difficult than I'd realized to be at ease in my body. I still felt the need to cover myself, chose clothes to hide behind. A long filmy shirt, sea green with a rope belt. A red peasant blouse with tiny mirrors sewn into the bodice. Flared jeans, hooded zip-up cardigans, a knee-length cable knit sweater that tied at the waist. Nothing clingy, nothing cropped.

Among my new clothes were two cashmere sweaters: a thigh length, raspberry turtleneck flecked with white angora, and a beige cowl neck. After so many years of coarse, brace-resistant fabric, their softness was a shock—cashmere on my neck where so recently metal had been.

In February a blizzard closed the schools for a week. The National Guard was called in to help clear away snow, and we couldn't open our front door against the drifts. Chipper and I stayed in my room listening to records, playing Scrabble, making up hard rock versions of soft rock songs on the acoustic guitar I was learning, badly, to play. We couldn't go anywhere; I may as well have stayed in my pajamas and robe, but every day I wore one of those two sweaters. My body had been going through the usual changes of puberty—hair and blood and odor—and the sweaters began to smell like something new, a yeasty smell, not unpleasant, but slightly distracting. I was becoming aware of my body in a different way, not as a thing to be withstood, but as a source of possible pleasure. And this frightened me. What obligations resided in the cashmere? What obligations had I been kept safe from? Touch me, the sweaters said, but I wasn't ready to be touched. I still had so much to learn.

When the blizzard ceased, when the drifts were cleared from our door, I went outside and lay down on my back, spreading my arms and legs to make snow angels. I was too old for this. I didn't care. All those years I couldn't. I swept my limbs back and forth, the snow so light and supple. I sank down into it, a creature more flesh and blood than she had ever felt before, imagining herself an angel.

I'll call him John. In truth I don't recall much about him, not even his name. Friend of a friend's boyfriend, something like that, he'd finished high school and was just hanging around. Most likely he had a job; how else to explain the car and the weed, neither of which were mine. The boy was not mine either; that is, I didn't think of him that way, although later I came to understand that, like the car and the weed, he thought of me as his.

We'd talked a few times at parties and once, with some other people in the car, he drove me home. So when he asked if I wanted to go to the beach and smoke some good weed it seemed like an okay idea. Better, anyway, than staying home watching reruns of *Mary Tyler Moore* and *Bob Newhart* with Chipper. I was nearly seventeen. None of the girls I knew were virgins. If I wanted to pass for one of them, those hair twirling, lip glossed girls who seem to know so much, I had some catching up to do. Only I wasn't at all sure what it was I wanted.

With the windows cracked I could smell the brine of low tide. He was rolling a fatty, one-handed, showing off. The radio must have been on because the radio was always on, Gregg Allman ramblin', Roger Daltrey leaving his girl behind, or, once in a while, a woman—Stevie Nicks, Linda Ronstadt—someone long-haired and plaintive. John and I shared a warm Rolling Rock. Other couples had come here to do the same thing and I could hear the music from their cars, smell their weed, see them making out. I'd known John a short while; he'd never seen me in a brace. I felt certain that had I been in one I would not have been in his car. Because of this I felt superior to him, the possessor of secret knowledge.

What had I supposed would happen when I said yes? On the one hand, I thought of my virginity as just another unwelcome difference. In theory I was blasé about sex, but I was skeptical about the enterprise as it applied to me personally, anxious about what it might entail.

John passed me the joint. I drew on it hard. He watched me smoke, as if expecting something. He was handsome, with black hair, light blue eyes, skin so pale I could see the threading of veins at his temples. For some reason their pulsing fascinated me. I took another hit. The song on the radio turned shrill and remote. Rainbow trails streamed from the headlights of passing cars.

I'm really stoned, I said, and John laughed and said, Yeah, I laced this with angel dust. Then he leaned in for a kiss.

Up close like that his teeth looked massive. His lips were salty and dry. His tongue fished about; I could feel the stringy tendon that attached it, clam-like, to the base of his mouth. He pressed against me, the muscles in his arms small and tight. I knew I was supposed to want him, or at least pretend that I did, placating him somehow, this boy who'd doped my dope, who thought that was an okay thing to do. But I didn't want him. The thing he'd done made me angry and scared. I pushed him away.

What? he said.

C'mon, he said.

Why'd you come here anyway if you don't wanna have fun?

I'm too stoned, I said. It's too much. Meaning the angel dust, meaning everything.

Maybe because the windows were open and there were other cars in the lot, because I could've yelled or tried to run or maybe because, at his core, there was a speck of decency in him, John finally gave up. He drove me to a girlfriend's house. We didn't speak on the ride there and I never saw him again.

Straddling

I no longer recall why I was in New York alone, that is without Chipper. Always before we'd traveled together, meeting our father on one of the subterranean platforms at Grand Central, then riding in his dark green sedan across town and down the FDR Drive to the East River high-rise he shared with two other divorced men. From the living room I could see the river, its tugboats and ferries and gulls all headed somewhere. I liked these New York weekends better than the ones we'd had in Bridgeport, with their enforced visits to his girlfriend's house, her four kids run amok, endless games of touch football and Capture the Flag. By the time my father moved to Manhattan, the girlfriend was gone. Instead of playing in her yard, we went to Italian street fairs or ate Chinese takeout—*Real Chinese, not that American chop suey crap you kids eat*—and if *Wide World of Sports* was on I'd read a book but mostly we watched movies on HBO, my father talking all through *Sleeper* or *Cabaret: Jesus this is some crazy stuff, you kids understand what's going on here?* To which I would always answer, yes.

I loved how New York contrasted with my quotidian life. Here was food I'd never tasted, people on the streets at night, apartments in the sky, pay phones set into red and green pagodas. Panhandlers, sidewalk musicians, a dancing chicken in a box. I had a sense that anything was possible. I pretended New York was my home.

It may have been, on this particular day, that Chipper had Little League. A fussy eater, he might not have wanted to waste an afternoon on strange foods. It's even possible that the occasion, a food festival in Central Park, was for me alone, a celebration of my newly acquired mobility. Eight months free of braces and casts, I was about to enjoy my first summer as a "normal" teenage girl, a girl unmarked by physical difference.

Be careful, my mother had warned and, to my father, You keep an eye on her. That summer the news coming out of New York was not good. Arson, crime, graffiti. A serial murderer who preyed on young women and called himself Son of Sam. Vigilante groups, subway muggings. The city was broken and broke.

Fifth Avenue did not look broke. We rushed past Cartier's, Tiffany's, Saks, my father keeping up a steady patter. *Jeez it's hot, you hungry sweetheart? Where we're going . . . every food in the world, you'll see, what're you now anyway, sixteen? Wow! My little girl, how'd you get so old?* Each word a stone in the wall between us. Charming and irrepressible and fun, a handsome man who sang in public and gave money to panhandlers, my father was everything Tom was not. Despite the pain he'd caused us, I wanted him to like me. But the clamor all around him—the girlfriends and roommates and other people's kids, the ringing phone and abrupt changes in plans—had always felt impossible to breach. He wanted not people so much as an audience. Now, alone with him for an entire afternoon, I was unsure what to say, how to act. I kept quiet to his torrent.

At Fifty-Ninth Street carriages lined the park's edge, the horses blinkered and bridled. I felt sorry for them. Still, I was excited. It was my first time in Central Park.

Once inside the gate my father seemed to relax. He let his shoulders sag. Food stalls had been set up on the lawn and he bought handfuls of tickets so we could have as much as we wanted, anything we craved. We ate voraciously, indiscriminately; we ate the way I read, going from burritos with salsa verde to hummus to garlicky Greek salads. For once I didn't care how much I ate. I wanted everything, all the foods and smells and noises in the park.

A few months later I would skip school to go to New York with Jimmy. The park that day would be mid-week serene and I would fantasize about living nearby. But on this afternoon there were jugglers, musicians, three-card Monte men and mimes. The grass was shiny, packed with people, late hippies and early punks and people like my father in suburban sportswear. A man in a ruffled yellow shirt played the steel drum. A dreadlocked man danced along, ecstatic, his hair streaming. I had the sense of being in a world apart, a bordered world, benign. At one stall a man was making banana daiquiris. My father bought two. We climbed a rock and sat in the sun, drinking the daiquiris, which were cold and sweet and mild. My father asked if I wanted some pie. Wait here, he said. I sipped my daiquiri and looked down at the people in the park. The sun was warm on my back and I felt drowsy and content.

From an adjacent rock a man came clambering over, a hippie-looking man, about twice my age, with a brown scruffy beard. By now I'd more or less outgrown my childhood fascination with hippies. To me the man looked dated, a relic. At first I didn't entirely grasp what he was doing on this rock—*my* rock—why he was pestering me, asking my name and how I was enjoying myself. I was not yet used to men noticing me. A year earlier I'd been invisible. Only the old women had noticed me, pausing to ask questions or say how sad. I was used to the old women, not the young men.

Partly I was flustered, partly annoyed, but mostly I felt apprehensive. Here I'd been enjoying myself when this man had appeared, demanding my attention, making me self-conscious. Should I flirt? Tell him to fuck off? Flatly, tersely, I answered his questions. *Yes I like the food, all the food, no I don't live in New York. My name? It's Patti.* And then I saw him, my father, bounding up the rock, a plate of pie in each hand and a terrible look on his face. Seeing it too, the man scurried off to try his luck on some other rock. My father boomed, loud enough for the man to hear, *Jesus Christ, I leave you alone for five minutes and look! Every weirdo in the park . . .*

Look at what? I wanted to answer because despite my discomfort I also knew that what had just occurred was ordinary enough, something I'd have to learn to navigate. And I was embarrassed in the way of a sixteen-year-old girl who had just been "rescued" by her father.

We ate our pie and left the park. The street was hot, unshaded, pulsing with too many bright things—taxis, buses, blinking signs: Walk and Don't Walk. The daiquiri had given me a buzz. A man in a wheelchair came pushing his way up Fifth Avenue, an obstacle course of pedestrians and vendors: pretzel and hot dog carts, sketch artists with easels, tourist groups, photographers hawking glossy skyline shots. People parted to let him pass. Slowly he guided his chair toward the park. I knew what he felt like, at least a little bit. The way your arms get tired, the way you're forced to look up at people who won't look back. A doctor had claimed that I might never walk again, but by the time I was using a wheelchair, post-surgery, I knew that was not true.

Suddenly I had to stop myself from crying. Not because I was happy or sad—I was neither of these things—but because the sense of my own autonomy, my freedom to move about in the world, was still so new I had difficulty believing it would not be snatched away.

I had one year left of school. To the hippie in the park I had no history. That was what I wanted, a blank slate. The year before had been something very different, and the following year would be different, too. Like Janus, Roman god of the new year, my gaze was fixed at once on the recent past and ahead toward the murky future. I longed to go unimpeded into that future, whatever that might turn out to be, but I feared being pulled back.

Gone

My mother arranged a trip to the Cape, just the two of us. We had three days, Tom's credit card, a hotel in Dennis Port. A reward, she explained, for all that lay behind. It was my last year at home; in the fall I would go to college in Boston.

On our first day away we wander the streets of Provincetown sharing a box of chocolate fudge, ruining our dinners. Even though I live in a beach town and love the ocean, I've spent so many years in seclusion from it that the sea air makes me feel slightly woozy, wanting to laugh at nearly everything: the bare-chested man with the snake around his neck, the patchouli and bong shops, the man in the dog collar. Here, I think, is a town where you can do what you want. I can do what I want now, too: go to the beach, take long showers, wear clothing I like, the remarkable recast as mundane. At a boutique my mother buys me a bikini, rust colored, with metallic stripes. Trying it on, adjusting the straps, tugging at the bottom, I am so taken by the newness of the experience, the liberation it represents, that I never consider the way the suit exposes my scar.

That night we go to a waterfront restaurant where my mother lets me order a glass of white wine. I've walked more than I'm used to walking, spent more time in the sun, and I feel sleepy and content, wishing every day could be like this one, with new things in it. And then, because I'm seventeen, I think why not? My mother is saying something about how much she'll miss me. First you, she says, then Chipper. Things between her and Tom have been more tense than usual. I can tell by the way she looks at him, the way he comes home from work and starts drinking, reading the paper with his feet up, waiting for her to make dinner even though she's worked all day too, stopping off to buy groceries or pick up his suits from the cleaners.

My mother butters a roll. Her hands could be my own; they are that similar to mine, that familiar. On her right pinky she wears a gold ring with a spiral pattern; her wedding band is unadorned. She has diamonds, special occasion jewelry she rarely wears. Still in her thirties, she is red-haired, Junoesque. Men have always loved her. Before she married Tom she had suitors, one of whom would send a dozen yellow roses to our house every week. In a strictly economic sense she has married well, far above the place she was born into. Because of this she has been able to give me things: the pink telephone and new bedroom furniture and stereo. She has, by her own admission, spoiled me.

I want to tell her that she's too good for Tom. She can leave him, get someone better. But even I know it's not that simple. Nothing's that simple when you come from nothing.

I'll miss you too, I say. And it's true, I know, I'll miss her like crazy. But there's something else I know which is that I do not want what my mother has—the house in the suburbs and the husband you put up with for the sake of kids who hate him, Sunday drives to aspirational homes, dinner at the same time each night. I know this the way a seventeen-year-old knows things, unequivocally. I'll miss you, I say, but already I'm thinking: Gone!

The woman on the album cover had her jacket slung over one shoulder, Frank Sinatra style. She wore a white shirt with torn off cuffs, a skinny black tie, unknotted, and a don't fuck with me expression. The songs she sang were about boy on boy rape, suicide, mythic birds, the birth of her baby sister. I'd never heard anything like it.

I'd discovered college radio and something was happening there. Gangly people with bad haircuts sang about buildings and lobotomies and politics, anything but romantic love. This was difference as indictment, as jerk and stutter and mismatched clothes. No one was bedroom poster ready. No one cared about pleasing anyone and that pleased me just fine.

I changed the way I dressed, adopting a thrift store, androgyne look. My uncle's dark green bomber jacket with a long black skirt. Men's T-shirts with pearls. Plastic shoes. Tom's old suit jackets and vests, ones my mother had picked out, not his usual polyester. Pinstriped wools, windowpane checks, a sky-blue seersucker blazer that I wore over a white cotton sundress, concealing my uneven shoulder blades. Twin City Discount, a Bridgeport warehouse, sold six-dollar stovepipe cords and holy medals that I safety pinned to my jacket lapels. A sartorial stoplight, I was making a statement about my sensibilities, not my body, which I kept malnourished, rattle-light.

My mother did not believe me when I said I wasn't coming back. She talked about the things we'd do together the following summer, restaurants we could go to now that I was old enough to be a viable dinner companion, plays and movies we might see. Maybe we'd take another trip, bring Chipper this time. I'd go to college, of course, live in a dorm, but I would return to Fairfield every summer, and during my winter breaks, and perhaps even for good once school was over. Those were her expectations.

The day after I turned eighteen I signed a lease on a basement apartment. For two months I'd been living in a dorm, a place I hated for its lack of privacy. The apartment was huge and close to school and my share of the rent, split between me and two friends, came to ninety-nine dollars. Because the radiators were attached to the ceiling pipes, a thing none of us had paid attention to during our brief pre-rental inspection, the apartment had virtually no heat. All that winter chunks of ice rained from the bathroom faucet. Mice raced around the kitchen at night. The windows opened onto the parking lot where a man sometimes slept in the dumpster. You had to peer inside before tossing out the trash. I could hear my upstairs neighbors fighting.

But none of this mattered, not really, because the apartment was more than a place to live; it was a way to assert my fledgling independence. Every time I thought about "home"—the boredom and sameness, Tom with his rages, my brother's sad cheerfulness, all the people I'd known since before I could remember, people who remembered too much about me, I knew I could not return. I had embarked on a life where no one knew me, a life where, quite literally, I had no back story. I could erase what had been simply by refusing to acknowledge it.

How much of this I grasped I'm not certain. I don't recall making a conscious decision to avoid speaking about the past. It just seemed irrelevant to my new circumstances. Past would not be prologue, so why bother bringing it up?

The lease signing took place in the manager's office, which he'd decked out to resemble a '70s era disco replete with red velvet barstools and mirror ball. His tobacco-stained dentures wobbled when he spoke. I could move in, he said, any time.

That night I called my mother from the dorm's pay phone to give her the good news.

You did what? she said. Who told you you could do that?

I'm eighteen, I replied. As if by turning the legal age for drinking and signing leases I'd somehow become able to support myself as well.

My mother was silent. I could hear crackling on the line. Behind me other girls waited to use the phone.

What the hell kind of place rents for ninety-nine dollars? she yelled. A whorehouse? A drug den?

I don't do drugs, I answered, indignant. And I'm not a whore. (That part, at least, was true.)

I won't send you any money.

Then I'll have to drop out of school.

It was an empty threat. Even if I meant it, which at the time I'm sure I did, who would hire an eighteen-year-old who lived in a ninety-nine dollar basement with no heat and a man sleeping outside her window in a dumpster? I'd have caved as soon as my savings ran out, a couple of months at best. My mother had to know this. But she also knew I was stubborn enough to at least make a show of living independently and that must have frightened her even more than the prospect of the whorehouse drug den basement. So she wrote me a check and came to Boston and took me shopping for dishes and blankets.

When are you coming home? she would periodically ask, to which I'd reply I'm already there. Not until years later did I consider how this must have pained her, how she must have felt she'd failed to make a home where her daughter felt at home.

Our lives had been so entwined, I'd been so dependent on her, that now, perhaps more than most people my age, I felt the need to break free. For my mother, however, this time in my life was a reward for all the hard work of caretaking. We'd live under the same roof. I'd be the companion who compensated for her bad marriage even as I was part of the reason for it. That much I did grasp and it made me want to flee.

Unchosen

Most Fridays he'd hock his guitar and we'd go to the movies or to Cafe' Algiers. During the week he'd pick up an extra shift waiting tables so he could get the guitar back in time to hock it again. Because my apartment was cold we spent weekends at his place, an attic in a house he shared with several other people, one of whom built robots in the basement. His bed was a futon on the floor; there was just enough space for that, his guitars, and a chest of drawers.

One afternoon we were eating lunch in a restaurant in Central Square, figuring out our plans for the night—what movie to see, who was playing at the Rat—when out of nowhere he asked about my personal relationship with Jesus. That was how he put it: What's your personal relationship with Jesus?

The way he phrased the question it sounded like an ad slogan. At first I thought he was joking. During the three months or so we'd been together the subject of religion had never come up. Nor did he look the part of a "Jesus freak," at least not as I imagined it, which had something to do with buzz cuts and high-water pants. Certainly not this vaguely hippie-looking man with his guitar and long blonde hair. Although having seen both *Godspell* and *Jesus Christ Superstar*, I probably should've known better.

We've never met, I said.

He scowled at me.

I'm serious, it's important.

Says who? I wanted to ask. With my fork I moved things around on my salad plate. Wherever this hairpin turn of a conversation was headed could not be good. My personal relationship with Jesus was something I'd spent zero time contemplating. I'd read the Beatitudes and liked their emphasis on social justice, but that was about all I knew. By dint of baptism I was Episcopalian. When my parents divorced, my mother found a friendlier congregation at my aunt's church, where we sang anti-war songs in the parish school's all purpose room. Friendly, that is, until my mother tried to enroll Chipper and me in Sunday School and was told that because we weren't Catholic we couldn't attend class, but she was welcome to buy the textbooks and teach us at home. And that was it for us and religion.

I don't have a relationship with Jesus, I said. Personal or otherwise. Why are we even talking about this?

He looked down at his sandwich remains for so long that I started to wonder if he was praying. When he looked up, his eyes were shiny and sad.

That's too bad, he said. Because Jesus is my personal savior.

What this meant, as far as I could tell, as far as he explained it to me in that Central Square restaurant with its steak sandwiches and iceberg lettuce salads, its fluorescent lighting and waitresses in white orthopedic shoes, the kind of place I felt out of place in, was that he wasn't really supposed to be having sex outside of marriage or, if he did, it wasn't supposed to mean anything. He needed to let me know that he could never love me, heathen that I was. We could still have fun together, don't get him wrong, but as far as anything more serious was concerned I shouldn't get my hopes up. Of course if I were to willing to change . . . And then he had to stop talking because I'd begun to choke on a piece of tomato from laughing so hard.

I don't love you either, I managed to sputter.

He looked stricken. What kind of woman was I, sleeping with a man I didn't love, laughing when he asked me about Jesus, choosing to reject him as her savior? Who knows what ideas about me he'd formed? Clearly they had little to do with the person sitting across from him. He could love me, maybe, if only I would become someone else. That afternoon I couldn't finish my lunch. I was too overcome, laughing.

He was the first man to ask me about the scar which, by the time I was twenty-four, was barely visible except at the base of my spine, where it widened slightly.

It's from an operation, I told him. Ten years ago. I had scoliosis.

Had. I remember marveling at this later, the cavalier way I consigned my scoliosis to the past. At the time, however, my answer seemed sufficient. Certainly it satisfied my questioner's curiosity, as he dropped the subject.

I spent the next decade with this man, my opposite in so many ways. A black man from Alabama, thirteen years my senior with two children from a previous marriage, he was a former semi-pro football player turned photographer, a dyslexic who disliked to read, a man confident to the point of entitlement, and so handsome that at first I found it difficult to look at him directly. In his presence I felt charmed, able to laugh off his joke about my funny walk, my "trick foot."

Early in our relationship he decided I could ride a bike, it was simple, anyone could do it. My inability had to be psychosomatic. He would teach me how.

I tried to explain that the issue was one of balance, not aptitude, but he refused to believe me. I just needed to try. And perhaps because I wanted to please him I convinced myself that maybe he was right. What fun it would be, after all, to ride along the Charles River, the breeze fanning my hair. I'd take my bike to work instead of the lumbering Mass. Ave. bus. We'd strap our bikes to the roof of his car and go on weekend trips. All I had to do was be a good pupil, something that came easily to me.

We walked his twelve-year-old daughter's bike to a scruffy neighborhood park, a patch of lawn littered with soda bottles, beer cans, dog shit. The day was cold for early fall, the park nearly empty. A couple of kids tossed a football around; an old man in a soiled overcoat sat on a bench drinking from a paper bag. The bike was pink with streamers on the handlebars. It did not look scary. But the moment I mounted it I knew I'd made a mistake.

Don't let go, I said. Promise you won't let go.

I promise. Just sit there, get used to it.

I felt dizzy. The ground looked far away. I didn't think this was a feeling I'd ever get used to.

Okay, he said. Ready?

He grabbed the handlebars. I kicked the kickstand free. The bike wobbled beneath me. He walked backward, leading. Then he let go with one hand. Instinctively I put my foot down.

What's wrong? You were doing great.

I was going to fall.

No you weren't. I had you.

You said you wouldn't let go. You promised.

I didn't let go.

I tried again and again. Each time he let go I toppled. Sometimes I righted myself, sometimes I landed in the grass, which felt surprisingly crunchy, not at all soft. The kids stopped playing and began to watch. At first they laughed, then they started shouting encouragement.

You gotta get your speed up, lady, one of them yelled. You gotta pedal faster.

Even the old man got involved, pointing and muttering between swigs.

Like to see you try it, I thought. We'll trade—I'll take the bottle and you get up on the bike.

I fell on my knees; I fell on my side. I fell with the bike on top of me. I chipped a fingernail, got dirt on my jeans, wiped out on a discarded Big Mac wrapper. Whenever I tried to get up a little speed I fell.

Everyone had advice. *Pedal faster. Don't look down. Just stay balanced.* But that—as I'd tried to explain—was the problem to begin with. I couldn't "just stay balanced."

Long after I was ready to quit I kept at it. I wanted to ride a bike. I really did. But I also knew that my stumbling was no more within my control than my boyfriend's stumbling over words whenever he tried to read. And did I bring home the paper every night insisting he attempt to read it? Did I quiz him on the contents?

His denial was a form of magical thinking. As if my failure, being a matter of choice, could with discipline be unchosen. The larger implication, of course, was that I couldn't possibly be satisfied with the way I was.

Yet to a certain extent that was true. While I had scant interest in the reclamation of my soul, and had broken up with the evangelical guitarist the day he tried to convert me, my body was a different matter. Given the option, a menu card at birth, I'd have checked the box for a straight spine. Perhaps then I'd have played sports, joined clubs, attended dances. Perhaps like Chipper and my parents I'd have been more social and self-assured. I might not have been so silent and aloof, might not have read quite so much, might not have begun turning myself into a writer right from the start. Who can say?

When I landed hands down in a pile of crusted dog shit I knew it was time to stop. Who was I trying to kid? I hadn't learned to ride a bike. I hadn't really thought I would. But I'd tried and in trying I'd shown my doubting companion what my words had failed to convey. I'd gone into the park the student and come out the teacher.

Backward Glances

And so. What was I then? What am I now? Formerly disabled? Healed? Reformed? (Literally, yes, I suppose this is so; I have been re-formed, pieced together with bone from my hips.) No one points, stares, yet I still can't shake the feeling that I'm "passing" for able-bodied.

At a conference not long ago I spoke as part of a panel on writing about disabilities. During the question and answer session a woman asked me about scarring. How has the notion of scarring influenced my work? Because I'd not given the issue much thought, her question intrigued me. Unlike some of the other disabilities represented on this panel—blindness, polio, Parkinson's disease—my scoliosis is not immediately apparent. Yet my scar, though concealed, brands me as "other," a member of some special non-elect. I struggled through an answer to her question, speaking about the reductive nature of disability, the dissonance inherent in hearing oneself described as a scar, a spine, how jarring this can be, especially for an adolescent, whose sense of identity has yet to jell. Only much later did I consider the question in terms of writing.

A book, Kafka said, should be an ice axe to break the frozen sea within us. Writing chips away at inauthenticity because for the work to matter it needs to get at what's essential. It's the thing that won't let go that counts. My own urge to write stems from a sense of vexation and inquiry: something is bothering me and I need to grasp why. Time, we know, does not heal all wounds. That's a fairy tale adage, something to see us through. Still, a certain amount of time needed to elapse before I felt able to write about any of this. The scar had to form, heal, fade. Until then I did not want to dwell. There are myths for this, too, cautionary tales for those tempted by the over-the-shoulder glance. Lot's wife. Orpheus. *Leave it alone. Don't look back.*

A few days after I turned forty, my father called to wish me a happy birthday. Decades earlier, during weekend visits, my father and brother had played games together. They wrestled on the carpeted floor. For Chipper there were love pinches, piggyback rides, Hungarian-sounding nonsense names. *Ignatz. Butchie Shondoke.* I was *Sweetheart.* I read and read. *Sweetheart we're going to toss the ball around, we'll be back, make yourself at home. Sweetheart, you like skiing? Jean-Claude Killy—watch this!* Later, when we were adults, Chipper—and only Chipper—was invited to my father's house on the New Jersey shore, a house I have never seen. I was my mother's daughter, my grandmother's pet: female, fragile, foreign. No place for me in this world of men. Fathers naturally favored their sons, their progeny, the person to carry on their names. This, at least, is how I had rationalized my father's preference.

He'd disappear. Months at a time; later, years. Stop answering phone calls, sending cards. Not even Chipper would know. Then a call, out of the blue. *I'm in town, business, your old man, he's got something cooking, let's have a drink.*

We stopped asking. This was normal, normal for us.

He'd stay in touch. Long enough so we'd think it just might last. Birthdays remembered, Christmases remarked. Gifts, cards, phone calls, drinks. Before dinner cocktails, dinner drinks, night caps. *One more nightcap, one for the road. Who wants another round? Your mother . . .* Here he would put down his highball glass, touch a knuckle to his eye. *Your mother's a fine woman. Terrific, the tops! But you need something, you call your old man. Got that? You Call Me!* Then he'd disappear again, leaving us to guess.

So when he phoned me, I was only mildly surprised, less that he'd called than that he'd remembered.

Your birthday! His tone was emphatic, his words slurred.

Two days ago.

Happy Birthday, sweetheart! Forty years old—wow! My little girl, forty. I can remember when you were just an itty bitty baby . . .

Oh, God, I thought. Oh, my God. This will go on all night.

Dad, listen, I have to . . .

. . . you were a little baby in your crib, so helpless, a little miracle just lying there. And I said God, let this be pure. Please, God, don't let this be corrupt.

Well that stopped me. I didn't know what to say. Who uses a word like "corrupt" to describe a newborn? Who invokes God, begging that an infant be "pure?" Somehow, instinctively, I understood that he was speaking not of me, but of Michael, his first child, the brother I'd never met. My father's love, his paternity, had been "corrupted" by his son's death, an event I'd never heard him mention.

The next day I told my mother about our conversation. Two months after my brother had died, my mother was pregnant again—with me. A bittersweet pregnancy, one imagines, fraught with sorrow, filled with hope. My mother had not yet learned to drive, and for weeks she'd been after my father to bring home the photos he'd taken of Michael before he'd contracted spinal meningitis: *a beautiful, healthy baby.* My mother told me the story: how my father hadn't wanted to develop the photos in the first place, how he demurred now, making excuses, quarreling. *Goddammit, I told you, I'm busy. I'll get to it!* Never saying what needed to be said—that he could not stand to look at photos of his dead son.

I can see them, my parents, married three years, still in their twenties, yet feeling so much older than their peers. My mother in a print house-dress, her auburn hair tied back with ribbon, dark crescents beneath her eyes. She's not been sleeping well. A winter afternoon; she's at the red linoleum table drinking Lipton's tea.

When she hears my father at the door does she rise? Does she bite her lip, smooth her hair? Earlier that day they'd quarreled again about the photos. She wants to see them, see her son, gone now three months.

My father storms into the kitchen. A large man, physically imposing. Snow on his belted overcoat, in his cropped black hair. He pulls the packet from his pocket, tosses it on the table. Here, he says, here are some photos of a dead baby!

Leave it alone. Don't look back. Like my brother, who confuses "mastectomy" with "vasectomy"—*Whatever, you know, I hate all those hospital words*—like so many others, my father has no words for illness, loss, or pain. He will not speak of it, not his father's death to lung cancer, nor his infant son's meningitis, nor, later, his mother's fatal stroke. Pressured by my grandmother, he came once to the hospital to see me, left within an hour, and did not return.

Language, of course, is not neutral. It fosters dichotomies, judgments. Sickness and health. Straight (straight arrow, straight and narrow path, straight shooter) and queer (queer duck, queer as a three-dollar bill, queering the deal . . .). Black and white. Disabled and able-bodied (. . . *being of sound mind and body I do hereby . . .*) I was on one side of the equation, then on the other. But the boundaries are porous. Each one of us is potentially disabled. Looking too closely at the other becomes a vexed act.

More than gender, it was illness that had always separated my father and me. Illness, frailty, death, loss. I was the replacement child, awkwardly formed, dangerous to love. Buffer between the son who had died and the robust boy, two years my junior, whom my father named for himself and whom my grandmother nicknamed Chipper because, she said, he was "a chip off the old block." My existence made it safe for him to be loved. It's taken me all of my life to understand this.

Legacy

In between classes I sip coffee in one of the university's Adirondack chairs, my face turned toward the sun. The lawns on this New England campus where I now teach are green and sloping, and the students, so close to semester's end, race down them, giddy with the knowledge that they will soon be set free. It's my favorite time of the school year.

I still find it mildly astonishing to be in this place. The first person in her immediate family to attend college. The great-grand-daughter of Hungarian immigrants who never fully learned English. The granddaughter of a woman who quit high school at age fifteen to support her family, and a man who'd been inter-mittently homeless as a boy. A woman whose mother chose her name for its many derivations. Pat, Patsy, Tricia, Patricia—I could change it to suit the surname of whomever I married. This was the world I was born into, a world in which women married young, stayed home raising babies if they were lucky, worked service jobs if they were not. When I accepted my first academic position, my mother said, I thought you were going to teach high school. I thought that's what you went back to school for.

I began to explain the difference between graduate degrees—MFA in English vs. MA in Education, the certification process for public school teachers, the import of a terminal degree. As I did so, my mother's face took on the fixed look of someone struggling to feign interest. So I switched tactics.

Well, I began, have you ever heard me say I wanted to teach high school?

No, but . . . I just thought that's what you wanted to do.

What my mother was not saying but was expressing nonetheless was her legacy, the paltry expectations she'd inherited and to some extent, despite herself, had passed down to me. It was a legacy that had prompted her to suggest I take courses in typing and shorthand so that I might have something to "fall back on" when luck and wits failed me. For despite having married a lawyer, I think she found it difficult to envision her children, or perhaps just her daughter, the member of some "elite" profession. The women in my family were secretaries, beauticians, nurses, clerks. They wore uniforms, changed bedpans, took dictation, painted other women's nails; often they stayed on their feet all day. I love every one of them. The men, whom I barely knew, joined the service; they worked in laundries or sold machinery or occasionally graduated to a middle management job.

Through hard work and luck I've managed to fashion a different sort of life. Unlike my grandmothers and aunt, I needn't spend days on my feet. Unlike my mother, I don't require a husband for financial support. And this is partly what I mean by luck—the luck of living in a time of expanded opportunities for women. The stamina my job requires is mental, not physical. No one cares whether professors can stand up straight, lift heavy boxes, touch their toes. My job demands that I read and write prodigiously, and I do so in a comfortable chair in the privacy of my bedroom. If I have chosen to become a member of the "cultural elite," it is because this is the club that's my natural home. And I can't help but wonder—how have my bones helped to put me here?

The facts are straightforward enough. I was awkwardly formed. In a world where popularity was linked to prowess I could not measure up. I walked funny, struck out at bat, toppled from my bike. I hid in my room; I read and wrote. Bound in brace and cast, I reimagined myself a writer, someone at ease in the library, the classroom, the book-filled study with its upholstered chair and ottoman, images I'd culled from *My Fair Lady* and the board game *Clue*. Writing helped me overcome a sense of physical inferiority;

it was a way to fight against the invisibility and isolation that attach to the disabled. With words I could reveal as much (or as little) of myself as I cared to even while my body remained concealed. Of course it is my nature, this indolence and bookishness. But bones helped sculpt my character, too, turning it inward.

Nature vs. structure, an unsolvable riddle. In the end there's really no way to know how much my misshapen body shaped me except to know that it did. My feelings about this body are likewise difficult to sort out. Indeed I may never untangle these strands—vexed from blessed, bitter from sweet.

Epilogue

This is not a redemption narrative. I leave those to the fairy tales, where what follows metamorphosis is a life of happily ever after. As a writer, I resist that ending, contravening as it does all we know about messy life. And it seems to me that one's former, unrehabilitated self can never entirely be effaced. Surely beauty, in the guise of a lovely lady, must harbor memories of beast, just as a butterfly retains the caterpillar's vestigial form.

Here is what happened to Dame Ragnell.

For five years she lived with Sir Gawain, who "never loved another woman so well." Then she died of unknown causes, leaving him bereft.

In *Flowers for Algernon*, that long ago book I read in ninth grade, the narrator undergoes an exquisitely painful moment during which he realizes he will shortly regress and die. Were these truncated lives a form of punishment for past sins, for residual ugliness and slowness? Most butterflies, we know, have a total life span of less than a year. Many years have passed since the events I describe took place. I am well into middle age, too old to die young. Yet so often the past feels more immediate than my quotidian present. A word, a look can bring back those years of difference.

I'm walking home from work, taking a shortcut through Boston's Copley Place Mall. Some kids are hanging out by a jewelry kiosk, drinking sodas, laughing. Seeing me, one of them yells, Hey, you walk just like Pee Wee Herman!

In grad school one winter there's a flu going around. I'm laid up for a week with fever, an ear infection, bronchitis. Because the bronchitis persists, the doctor on call at university health services wants to x-ray my lungs. There on film are my ghostly ribs, the daunting "S" of my spine, the rods that hold everything together.

The doctor whistles, as though impressed.

Wow, he says, you've got scoliosis up the butt!

I go for a mammogram and the technician, frustrated that I cannot bend into the machine the way she needs me to, has begun repeating herself. Like this, she says, arcing her own supple body far to the left. I've already explained about my spinal fusion, explained that what she wants is impossible for me. Like this! She tries to wrench me into position.

What are you doing? I knock her hands away. You could injure me.

The expression on her face is one I recognize whenever I explain to a student why, after missing three week of classes, it is no longer possible to pass the course. Incomprehension and shock.

You're crooked, she says. I'm trying to help you stand up straight.

I lower the hospital gown, show her my scar.

You need to bend, she says.

Central Park, I'm alone. I've been writing and need to take a break. On the path by the Harlem Meer, a man cuts toward me. I change sides, trying to walk around him, but he blocks my way. He looks enraged, unbalanced. I know that look and the way a certain kind of woman, alone and indifferent to the male gaze, can incite fury in a certain kind of man. My adrenaline is up; my heart feels loud. What does he want? How can I get past him?

You walk like a God damned turtle, he sputters. What's wrong wit chu? Huh? What the fuck is wrong wit chu?

He waves his arm wildly then, his anger apparently spent, he continues on his way.

I've just bought my wedding dress, sleeveless beige silk, knee-length, with lace at the top and a high bodice, nearly an empire waist, which will require some assistance from a new bra. This specialty shop on the Upper West Side has everything: sports bras, push-ups, and strapless of course, but also bullets, mini-mizers, racerbacks, convertibles, hook extenders, and something called "cleavage cupcakes" that I do not ask about. Still, the salesgirl has trouble fitting me. She brings maybe half a dozen selections, some of them lovely, none of them fitting quite right. In desperation, she finally calls in an older associate, a buxom woman who looks so much like my grandmother that I can't help picturing her in a robe with a Manhattan in one hand and a smol-dering Newport in the other.

Nothing fits, the salesgirl moans. She's lopsided.

The older woman sucks in her breath. She gives the girl a withering look. They fit for prostheses at this shop, they fit women with mastectomies, they have bras in sizes AA to JJ. The non-conformist body is their business. I can just about imagine the upbraiding that will take place when I am gone. *We do not—repeat do not—call our customers lopsided. Have I made myself clear?*

Like the older woman, I want to be formidable. Who is this girl to comment on my shape? What the hell does she know? But for whatever reason, I'm just not up to the task.

It could be that word—"lopsided"—how it makes me think of lollipops, the sweet comfort of them after childhood visits to the pediatrician. Or perhaps it's my new dress and the occasion it represents. Or maybe I'm becoming inured. Strangers will have their say. The girl, I sense, is well meaning enough. And unlike the doctor or the technician, she has no real power. There is nothing she can withhold.

Remember? Do you remember how we'd stay up all night, go to clubs, after hours parties, show up for class in the morning not even tired? Amazement in her voice.

This woman, my best friend, is a model of industry. We've known each other practically all of our lives. In college she'd been a dancer and her posture is still regal. Both she and her husband are athletic; they run, hike, play tennis, ride their bikes all over New York. Among other things, Carey has renovated two homes, a brownstone in Harlem and a gutted building in the East Village. She's built a house in upstate New York, started a community development corporation, and helped to create affordable housing in post-Katrina New Orleans where, as a hobby, she'd constructed makeshift bus shelters because she couldn't stand seeing old women waiting on the sidewalk in the sun. All this while caring for a one-hundred-and-two-year-old aunt in the South Bronx.

Who are you kidding? I say. You do more now in a day than we did during an entire week back then. Maybe an entire semester.

It's true, she concedes. But these days by eleven o'clock all I want is to go to bed.

Tonight, well past eleven, we are celebrating. A prestigious new job for Carey and my marriage, two days earlier, in the living room of her Harlem home.

Like me, my new husband is thin, small-boned; "your twin," people have joked, and I think it is true, the way so many couples resemble each other, the narcissism of love. Unlike me, he is a former athlete, a runner and soccer player, quick moving, a good dancer, light on his feet. He has never spent a night in the hospital, never had anything physically wrong. His diagnosis of leukemia is four months away. Soon there will be DNA tests, white blood cell counts, CT-Scans, a bone marrow biopsy. His arm will bruise from the needles as mine once did and, like me, he will become dependent on others for his care. His appearance too will change, marking him. Cold sores, an enlarged spleen, lymph nodes so swollen he will be unable to button the collars of his dress shirts. He will go through pneumonia, shingles, a month long bout of flu, then six months of chemotherapy that will finally send him into remission, a remission I will never entirely trust, one that keeps me mindful of the Fates, those grim sisters with their thread and tape measure and scissors. Exhausted, he will make jokes to cheer me, mimicking that peasant in *Monty Python and the Holy Grail*: "I'm not dead yet!" He will endure. And whenever he tells me how frightened he feels, how vulnerable in his hospital gown, I will do the only thing that makes sense to me, which is to hold him and say, "I know."

But tonight we do not know. Tonight we've come to the Lenox Lounge for open mic. A huge woman in a tiara and electric blue gown has arrived too late to get on the performance list. She screams at the emcee, the aptly named Patience, calls him a "fuckin' motherfucker!" threatens to "tear the place apart" before she is escorted out. No one here is shy. Obese women, bald paunchy men, skinny hipsters, a diva or two, a Japanese girl with acne; good, bad, mediocre, they each get up to perform. I watch, fascinated. What makes people so unabashed? When the house band kicks in and Patience takes up the sax, the room really starts to swing. But by then Carey needs to go home.

It's the PMS, she says. The PMS and the job—she just can't stay up so late anymore—and the PMS. My breasts are killing me, she says. I feel like I weigh a ton. Her husband says he will walk her home and come back to join us; we should order him another drink. Again Carey apologizes.

You ever feel so uncomfortable in your body that it's like you're in some foreign space? she asks. It used to do everything I wanted, and now it won't. It's frustrating, you know what I mean?

Yes, I say, yes I do. I know all about that feeling.

Trick foot, Pee Wee Herman, "scoliosis up the butt." The comments still sting. Their subtext is clear: you are an alien in the realm of the able-bodied, holding no passport here.

Unlike my athletic friend, however, I will stay for the set. I will walk home unassisted; will walk, in fact, over the Brooklyn Bridge and back to help raise money for blood cancer research.

My body will never do everything that I desire. It will never permit me to swim great distances, ski the Alps, bike the French countryside, skate in Central Park. But it does a lot more than I'd once thought possible.

You have the bones of a seventy year old, my doctor had said. Yet they support me, these geriatric bones. In their own crooked way, and despite my neglect, they hold me up. They are, in no small sense, miraculous.

About the Author

Patricia Horvath's stories and essays have been published widely in literary journals including *Shenandoah, The Massachusetts Review, New Ohio Review, The Los Angeles Review, Confrontation*. She is the recipient of New York Foundation for the Arts Fellowships in both fiction and literary nonfiction and the Goldenberg Prize for Fiction at *Bellevue Literary Review*. She teaches at Framingham State University in Massachusetts.

Books from Etruscan Press

Lines of Inquiry | H. L. Hix
Rain Inscription | H. L. Hix
Shadows of Houses | H. L. Hix
Wild and Whirling Words: A Poetic Conversation | Moderated by H. L. Hix
Art Into Life | Frederick R. Karl
Free Concert: New and Selected Poems | Milton Kessler
Who's Afraid of Helen of Troy: An Essay on Love | David Lazar
Parallel Lives | Michael Lind
The Burning House | Paul Lisicky
Quick Kills | Lynn Lurie
Synergos | Roberto Manzano
The Gambler's Nephew | Jack Matthews
The Subtle Bodies | James McCorkle
An Archaeology of Yearning | Bruce Mills
Arcadia Road: A Trilogy | Thorpe Moeckel
Venison | Thorpe Moeckel
So Late, So Soon | Carol Moldaw
The Widening | Carol Moldaw
Cannot Stay: Essays on Travel | Kevin Oderman
White Vespa | Kevin Oderman
The Dog Looks Happy Upside Down | Meg Pokrass
The Shyster's Daughter | Paula Priamos
Help Wanted: Female | Sara Pritchard
American Amnesiac | Diane Raptosh
Human Directional | Diane Raptosh
Saint Joe's Passion | JD Schraffenberger
Lies Will Take You Somewhere | Sheila Schwartz
Fast Animal | Tim Seibles
One Turn Around the Sun | Tim Seibles
A Heaven Wrought of Iron: Poems From the Odyssey | D. M. Spitzer
American Fugue | Alexis Stamatis
The Casanova Chronicles | Myrna Stone
Luz Bones | Myrna Stone
The White Horse: A Colombian Journey | Diane Thiel
The Arsonist's Song Has Nothing to Do With Fire | Allison Titus
The Fugitive Self | John Wheatcroft
YOU. | Joseph P. Wood

Etruscan Press is Proud of Support Received from

Wilkes University

Youngstown State University

The Ohio Arts Council

The Stephen & Jeryl Oristaglio Foundation

The Nathalie & James Andrews Foundation

The National Endowment for the Arts

The Ruth H. Beecher Foundation

The Bates-Manzano Fund

The New Mexico Community Foundation

Drs. Barbara Brothers & Gratia Murphy Fund

The Rayen Foundation

The Pella Corporation

The Raymond John Wean Foundation

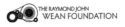

Founded in 2001 with a generous grant from the Oristaglio Foundation, Etruscan Press is a nonprofit cooperative of poets and writers working to produce and promote books that nurture the dialogue among genres, achieve a distinctive voice, and reshape the literary and cultural histories of which we are a part.

etruscan press

www.etruscanpress.org

Etruscan Press books may be ordered from

Consortium Book Sales and Distribution
800.283.3572
www.cbsd.com

Etruscan Press is a 501(c)(3) nonprofit organization.
Contributions to Etruscan Press are tax deductible
as allowed under applicable law.
For more information, a prospectus,
or to order one of our titles,
contact us at books@etruscanpress.org.